M000025052

HOW TO KILL CANCER CELLS

Make Your Body Healthy Now

Natalie Mitchell

Cancer Prevention Coach

The information in this book is based on the experience and research of the author. It is not intended as a substitute for consulting with your physician or other health-care provider. Any attempt to diagnose and treat an illness should be under the direction of a health-care professional. The publisher, author and editor are not responsible for any adverse effects or consequences alleged to result or resulting from the use of any of the suggestions, preparations or procedures discussed in this book.

ISBN: 9780988538719

Published by Accretive Solutions Ltd

Mail: PO Box HM 2190, Hamilton HMJX, Bermuda

www.cancercells.info

contact@cancercells.info

Editor: Colin Barnes

March 2013

HOW TO KILL CANCER CELLS

Make Your Body Healthy Now

Natalie Mitchell

Cancer Prevention Coach

CONTENTS

This book is dedicated to the memory of Constance Barnes.

"People generally achieve magnificent things when their backs are up against the wall and they are forced to tap into the wellspring of human potential that lies within them."

Robin Sharma

INTRODUCTION

Quite naturally, many of us fear cancer and worry that we may already have the disease or that we are someday going to suffer from it. All of us wish to reduce the chance that we will suffer from cancer at some stage of our lives. Fortunately, there really is much that each one of us can do to control the threat of cancer in our lives. This book will explain how, through an acquired knowledge of, and a greater understanding about, the root causes of the disease, we can take effective, consistent actions which are completely in our control, to avoid cancer developing in our body during our lifetime.

My name is Natalie Mitchell and I became driven to write this book for you as a result of the force of numerous motivating experiences in ten plus years of my work with many cancer and chemotherapy patients as they journeyed with their fight to recover from cancer. Too often I worked to help cancer sufferers maintain a level of strength and vitality through their chemotherapy course and afterwards. Until they received a cancer diagnosis, almost without exception, they had no idea how their past diet and stress had contributed to the unfortunate success of the cancer cells in their body having been allowed to develop to the point that their body's natural defense capabilities were overwhelmed and unable to neutralize the growth of the cancer cells fueling the disease within their bodies.

With the additional knowledge support from study of much well-established and confirmed medical and scientific cancer research over the last century as well as being a constant student myself of cancer cell behavior, I feel very strongly that I should now make vital cancer cell information available to all who want to be proactive in their quest to remain healthy and free from cancer.

I go into some detail about a core piece of knowledge about cancer avoidance which is the understanding that we, as individuals, can deny cancer the type of internal body environment in which cancer cells find nourishment to grow and multiply.

I also feel it is important to share with my readers an understanding of what cancer cells feed on and what their favorite foods are so the reader, armed with this knowledge, can confidently deprive the cancer cells in their body of the fuel they seek in order to multiply on the scale they need to become destructive to our body tissue and organs.

The statistic below explains why we are all so much more cognizant today of the cancer threat to our bodies:

"In 1904 only 1 out of 24 Americans had cancer in their lifetime. Today the cancer rate is 1 out of 2 for men and 2 out of 3 in women."

The clear conclusion is that people in 1904 were much healthier than we are today.

What were they or their bodies doing differently?

Simply put, much of the food most of us enjoy today is not healthy for our bodies and does not meet the needs of our internal cells, organs and tissues for them to function normally year after year. As you will learn in more detail throughout my book, the root cause of increasing global cancer rates is the increasing level of acidity in the modern diet. There are several contributing causes for high acidity in our bodies. Compared with the diet of people a hundred years ago, the modern day diet in growing numbers of countries contains a high percentage of processed foods of all kinds. Processed foods are typically high in acidity creating ingredients such as sugar and white enriched flour. Other frequently consumed contributors to a state of high acidity in the body are soda drinks, refined carbohydrates, meat, cheeses, and alcohol. Processed foods have low alkalinity levels which is absolutely the opposite to the alkalinity levels in natural foods people predominantly consumed a century ago such as green vegetables, fresh fruits, spices, etc. Unfortunately, with our high processed food intake, we are literally being pumped full of food additives such as high fructose corn syrup, refined flours, sugar, and artificial sweeteners – all of which are extremely acidic to the human body.

Sound medical research and study stretching back to cancer disease discoveries beginning as early as the last century support much of the knowledge you are about to read in this book. To give you an example, **Dr. Otto Warburg, as early as 1924,** was able to determine that cancer cells are not oxygen breathing and that they have an anaerobic condition. The relevance of this is core to today's cancer avoidance.

While our doctors of medicine and contemporary medical science are doing their best for us when it comes to cancer diagnosis, there continues to be constant research about the different types of cancer, as well as into many other life threatening illnesses, in terms of how best to treat cancer patients and improve cancer survival rates.

It is clear however, that too little is being done from a research perspective within societies in general to understand how humans can avoid cancer in the first place. In spite of better medical science and treatment, humans are still getting cancer at a faster rate than ever. I firmly believe that mankind will be better off spending more research money to fully understand the cause of cancer, particularly through cancer causing agents in the world we live in, rather than on how to treat the effect of it on the body by which time it is already at a quite advanced stage of development and at its most difficult to cure.

I have learned that most cancer sufferers have unfortunately never had access to the knowledge you will find in this book about nurturing your body to allow it to stay cancer free and making a real difference to your chances of avoiding cancer in your lifetime. This knowledge is also of great power and relevance if you do get cancer, in terms of successfully becoming cancer free again. Yes, know that cancer does not need to be a terminal disease.

I was driven to write this book because there is so much that we, as individuals, can do for ourselves every day of our precious lives to prevent our bodies from succumbing to serious illness, including cancer. While everybody on our beautiful planet Earth is born with cancer cells in their body, fortunately not everybody develops cancer. You are probably wondering why many people remain cancer free even as you recognize the statistics showing increasing numbers of people diagnosed with many different forms of cancer.

It may astound you that even with the medical technology available nowadays doctors can only diagnose cancer disease when people already have developed **BILLIONS of active cancer cells** in their body.

You will be very interested to learn, therefore, that your every day decisions on what foods to put into your body will effectively determine during the course of your life, whether or not cancer cells stay dormant and even get destroyed by your body's defenses while your healthy cells remain perfectly happy.

More about this and the specifics a little bit later in the book and most importantly, I would like you to feel greatly encouraged and motivated to learn as I explain to you in the chapters ahead that there is indeed so very much you can DO every day in the choices you make for your body to sustain it in a healthy, cancer free state. It is so important my dear reader, never to forget you are, in fact, the Master of your Body, Mind and Spirit. This is an awesome responsibility that so many of us take for granted with hardly a thought.

You are the ONE who decides and acts on what to feed your precious body with. The more you are aware about how much real and effective control you can actually have over your body's health by reading this book, the more power and knowledge you will gain from these pages to apply the right decisions and choices for achieving a state of sustained health in the years ahead. The more informed actions and decisions you take in the future will improve the quality of your life in so many different ways as good health is the foundation for success and happiness in all aspects of life as well.

Our body is an amazing, complex factory where all organs are interdependent with each other in order to give us the health that often we take for granted. Our immune system acts as our body's defensive mechanism and will function perfectly well if provided with the appropriate body environment to fight in! As much as 70% of your immune system cells are found in your gut. You can readily make the connection between the quality of your food and your health!

In the chapters ahead I will inform you, step by step, how you can improve your health to avoid cancer, how to enhance your energy level, as well as the sharpness of your brain and memory capacity - from whatever stage you are at right now.

The most important thing is that you are here and reading this book so you are on your way to giving yourself the incredible opportunity to acquire and apply the knowledge you are going to learn in the chapters below, every day from today, the beginning of the rest of YOUR healthy life! Reading my book will give you lifelong tools to tremendously improve the quality of your life and you will start experiencing your health and energy level improving in quite a short period of time if you can follow the advice with a sustained level of diligence and continuity. As you know there is only one thing on this planet, which is impossible to buy or replace, and this is your body's HEALTH! It requires the right knowledge, motivation and most importantly, the concrete actions on your part, which you should have confidence in carrying out, knowing how relevant and effective your choices will be to the degree of health that you enjoy for the rest of your life.

You will also gain an understanding of how the powerful combination of appropriate Nutrition, positive thinking, positive emotions and **actions** can deeply influence how resistant our bodies can be to different illnesses. Interestingly, there are many case histories of identical twins where one twin remains perfectly healthy through life and the other twin develops a serious disease. I see our body as a very intelligent and complex factory created by God and while its complexity does not prevent it sometimes being damaged by cancer cells, it always will respond and do everything it can to cure and **heal itself** provided it is given the necessary environment to do so.

For you to be most successful, it will require your dedication to make changes to your diet no doubt and for you to continually reinforce your positive attitude toward nurturing your precious life. With this book, you have everything you need, at your fingertips, to make a difference. It is all in your hands now as you are the caretaker of your precious Mind, Body and Spirit. The knowledge I accumulated, which I am so happy to be sharing with you, has already helped many people that share your desires and much of this knowledge, which unfortunately has not been widely known, has been used successfully for centuries. Fortunately, much of this knowledge became known to me in my studies over the years. You will now use this knowledge as well and what a great gift to your health and well being your commitment to help yourself will be! **Investing in acquiring and then using the knowledge to help your body cells may be the best investment you can ever make!** Let's start this journey together as I am here to help you understand what your blood cells would tell you right now **if they could speak to you.**

Chapter 1

Creating the Environment Within Your Body To Kill Cancer Cells.

*"He who has a **why** to live for, can bear any **how**."*

Friedrich Nietzsche

*"We delight in the **beauty** of the **butterfly**, but **rarely acknowledge** the **changes** it has gone through **to achieve that beauty**."*

Maya Angelou

Let me first explain the nature of cancer cells and what causes them to become active or inactive in the tissues of the human body. It is not a well-known fact that everyone on Planet Earth has cancer cells in their body - we do, we are born with them. What we must recognize is that cancer cells only become active and a threat to our tissues and organs when an acidic environment in our bodies has developed from the foods we have consumed. An acidic body environment allows the cancer cells to multiply and grow. Once we understand that our bodies' susceptibility to cancer is directly connected to the food that it has been given to consume, we must also recognize that our bodies are hugely influenced by what kinds of food and drink we put in them and that this is true not only with respect to our resultant physical body weight but also to the conditions existing in our internal organs. Understanding the significance and relevance of nourishment choices, we can then focus our food and nutrition knowledge toward providing our body with the support it needs to effectively use its natural defensive systems to remove and prevent active cancer cells existing within.

By controlling the cancer cell environment in our body every day, month, year of our lives, through the nutrition we give it, we can beat and prevent cancer!

Every human has cancer cells in their body and it is not in itself something you should worry about. You will read the material in this book and going forward, will be equipped with the necessary knowledge to apply to your precious body and mind regarding lifelong management of cancer as a threat to your health. The danger of cancer disease starts when otherwise passive cancer cells start multiplying rapidly in the body. For cancer cells to do that, an acidic environment has to have developed in the body and the food cancer cells thrive on has to be present.

As I indicated in the Introduction, it is surprising but true that cancer cells do NOT show up in the typical modern diagnostic test results until they have multiplied **to a few BILLION active cancer cells** in the body. It takes years for them to reach this number. Some people think that cancer appears so suddenly in the human body, in fact, billions of cancer cells don't usually appear suddenly but over considerable periods of time.

If we allow an acidic environment to persist in our system day after day, month after month, year after year, the cancer cells will be incentivized to MULTIPLY.

Let's take a further look at what research is telling us about the state of the human body when it is diagnosed with cancer.

Research has proven that terminal cancer patients can have an acidity level 1,000 times greater than normal healthy people. An **acidic** body is a body that is highly vulnerable to cancer disease. Research has proven that the disease cannot survive in an alkaline body state in contrast to the disease's ability to thrive in an acidic environment.

The basic truth and therefore an important piece of knowledge to understand and accept is that our bodies simply cannot fight diseases if our body pH is not properly balanced to an alkaline state. An **acidic body** becomes a **magnet** for over 150 diseases like cancer, diabetes, multiple sclerosis, arthritis, heart disease, gall and kidney stones, and many more.

In detail, as this is so really important for you to understand and use effectively to empower and strengthen your body's defensive mechanisms, I am now going to spend some time explaining how you can deprive your cancer cells of the acidic environment within your body that they will thrive on if given the opportunity.

First, as to the important question of why some tissues in the body become prone to cancer, it is helpful to understand the nature, causes and effects of tissue **acidity** and **alkalinity** levels and how critical this is to the natural body defensive mechanisms our cells and tissues rely on.

Cancer prone tissues are those that have become more **acidic**, whereas **healthy tissues** remain within the normal **alkaline levels that the body works at delivering to cells and tissues**. Optimum alkalinity levels also depend on **correct oxygen levels in the body, which help to neutralize acidity**, while, conversely, abnormal acidity levels prevent oxygen from reaching the tissues that need it. When tissues become devoid of free oxygen, acidity levels rise within the tissue which can then activate otherwise dormant cancer cells.

A body in a state of Alkalinity allows oxygen into the body's tissues. The most important task you will be focusing on with the knowledge you find in this book is how to create and maintain a **more alkaline environment** in your body, consistently, over time, in fact, for Life! You will learn how you can continuously nurture this alkaline environment so that your body makes and keeps **cancer cells inactive**.

The way I explain this in more detail, is to talk in terms of the significance of the relationship between the pH level of the body and of the pH level of the different foods that we put into our bodies. Relative to what our bodies required pH levels are, you will understand which foods have higher **alkalinity** values and therefore more **cancer beating power** for our blood cells and tissues than those foods which are more acidic and which, if allowed to continue to be part of our normal diet, will allow cancer cells to continue to be active and potentially multiply.

The pH scale measures how acidic or alkaline a substance is and ranges from 0 to 14, with 7.0 being the neutral state. For this discussion, body pH readings below 7 are **acidic** and above 7 are considered **alkaline**.

You are probably wondering what your body's healthy state pH level should be and what it is currently.

Medical science has determined that blood, lymph and cerebral spinal fluid in the human body are designed to be, and stay healthy in, an alkaline environment at a pH level of <u>7.4 or higher</u>.

"At a pH level slightly above 7.4 cancer cells within our body become dormant and at the more alkaline level of pH 8.5, cancer cells will actually die while healthy cells will live" (Barefoot, pages 66-67).

This knowledge has given rise to the development of a variety of nutritional based regimens designed to increase the alkalinity of the body's tissues through:

1. The intake of more alkaline **vegetarian foods;**

2. The drinking of alkalizing **fresh fruit and vegetable juices and;**

3. The intake of foods particularly rich in **alkaline minerals** including **calcium**, **potassium**, **magnesium**, **caesium**, **rubidium, sodium, and selenium** as well as **antioxidant vitamins**.

I hope you are now at a point where you are really excited that you have, within your grasp, the developing knowledge and motivation to power your body to a steady state of cancer free health. You should now commence, as soon as possible, taking the steps to help your body to **become alkaline** and to **stay that way** so that your blood cells and tissues actually **have the power to neutralize the cancer cells in your body**.

How you will achieve this - by understanding what kind of foods create the most and the least acidity in the body - you are going to learn from the detailed information in my book. You can now appreciate that you should immediately start and continue eating daily more foods that have pH levels higher than neutral 7, while permanently eliminating foods, with few exceptions, from your diet that have pH levels of less than 7. When a body is full of acidity, the body cells and tissues consume a lot more **energy** to **deal with the acidic state, which is** why so many people experience **fatigue**, **lack of energy** and even **depression**.

Your best help for your body will result from your devotion to a focused daily regimen of buying, cooking and eating the right "alkaline" foods to allow your body to disarm your cancer cells and put them into "hibernation" permanently.

Incredibly, much of the food we like and find in our local grocery store is actually dangerously acidic to our body's tissues. While processed foods are generally highly acidic, it is surprising but true that even natural foods can be too acidic for our bodies. Who would have expected for example, that **oranges that taste so delicious and which are so universally popular,** have a pH level of **3.69 - 4.34,** which in fact is <u>very acidic.</u> The same circumstances are true with many people's favorite - tomatoes, particularly those that are eaten before they are **fully ripened**.

You may now be at the point where you will want to commit to helping your system every day to discourage cancer cells from activating in your body as much as possible. **The tables you will read below will allow you to be clearly and quickly informed about, and** to make the decision to **avoid today and every day,** the vegetables and fruits that do not help the body stay within its normal alkalinity range. Your blood cells are craving for you to give them a healthier environment and you can totally satisfy their needs once you have studied the information on acceptable and unacceptable foods contained in this book.

I am sure you are by now worrying that perhaps your diet will become boring and tasteless. Well, I have good news for you. We can make and keep your system **optimally alkaline** by enabling you to replace the **acidic foods** in your diet with foods that are **alkaline as well as being delicious to your taste buds.** You can start helping your body today with delicious alternatives to select from which will allow you to continue to enjoy your food every day!

Some "borderline" neutral pH vegetables and fruits are acceptable to eat when they are fully ripe and grown organically and this is indicated opposite each one in the table below. Later, I will also explain why it is so important for you to consume **organic** alkaline foods as much as possible and most probably you already know some of the reasons.

Earlier I mentioned the importance of foods rich in alkaline minerals. Here is a quote from Dr. Warburg and Dr. Brewer's research that shows the importance of alkaline minerals and how they work within cancer cells.

*"A mass spectrographic analysis of cancer cells showed that the cell membrane readily attached **caesium, rubidium and potassium**, and transmitted these elements with their associated molecules **into the cancer cell**. In contrast cancer membranes did not transmit sodium, magnesium, and calcium into the cell: the amount of calcium within a cancer cell is only about 1% of that for normal cells. **Potassium** transports glucose into the cell. **Calcium** and **magnesium** transport **oxygen** into the cell. As a consequence of the above, **oxygen cannot enter cancer cells** so the glucose which is normally burned to carbon dioxide and water undergoes fermentation **to form lactic acid** within the cell."*

Dr Warburg pointed out this anaerobic condition, **as early as 1924.**

*"**Potassium** and especially **rubidium** and **caesium** are the most basic of the elements. When the cancer cells take them up they will thus **raise the pH of the cells**. Since they are very strong bases as compared to the **weak lactic acid** it is possible that the pH will be raised to values in **the 8.5 to 9 ranges**. In this range **the life of the cancer cell is short**,*

*being a matter of **days** at the most. The **dead cancer cells** are then absorbed by the body fluids and eventually eliminated from the system."* – **Dr Brewer.**

Medical research has found that cancer grows slowly in a **highly acid body environment** (because the **acids** cause it to **partially** destroy itself) and may actually grow more quickly as your body becomes more alkaline **prior to** reaching **the healthy pH slightly above 7.4 where the cancer cells become dormant.**

Therefore, you will want to raise your **pH above 7.4 as quickly as possible** by every means available. Once you have achieved a pH above 7.4, it is useful to monitor your saliva and urine pH regularly to ensure that your body remains **sufficiently alkaline**.

It is important to understand that we are not talking about stomach acid or the pH of the stomach. Here we are talking about the pH of the body's fluids and tissues, which is an **entirely different matter**.

The Saliva PH test is a simple test you can do to measure your susceptibility to cancer, heart disease, osteoporosis, arthritis, and many other degenerative diseases. Buy your Saliva pH test kit from your local drug store or pharmacy.

Please don't worry if your saliva test shows too much acidity as I am going to provide you with all necessary tools to enable you to alkalize your system as soon as possible.

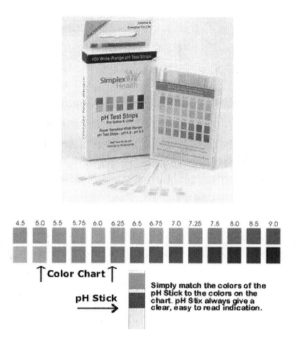

How to Perform the Saliva pH Test

First, you must wait at least 2 hours after eating. Fill your mouth with saliva and then swallow it. Repeat this step to help ensure that your saliva is clean. Then after the third swallow, put some of your saliva onto the **pH paper**.

The pH paper should turn blue. This indicates that your saliva is slightly alkaline at a healthy pH of 7.4. If it is not blue, compare the colour with the chart that comes with the **pH paper**. If your saliva is acid (below pH of 7.0) wait two hours and repeat the test.

"When healthy, the pH of blood is 7.4, the pH of spinal fluid is 7.4, and the pH of saliva is 7.4. Thus the pH of saliva parallels the extra cellular fluid...pH test of saliva represents the most consistent and most definitive physical sign of the ionic **calcium and other alkaline minerals and antioxidant vitamins deficiency syndrome**...The pH of the non-deficient and healthy person is in the 7.5 (dark blue) to 7.1 (blue) slightly alkaline range. The range from 6.5 (blue-green), which is weakly acidic to 4.5 (light yellow) which is strongly acidic, represents alkalinity states from mildly deficient to strongly deficient, respectively.

Most children are dark blue, a pH of 7.5. Over half of adults are green-yellow, a pH of 6.5 or lower, **reflecting the calcium and other alkaline minerals and antioxidant vitamins deficiency** of aging and lifestyle defects. **Cancer patients are usually a bright yellow, a pH of 4.5**, especially when terminal." The Calcium Factor: The Scientific Secret of Health and Youth, by Robert R. Barefoot and Carl J. Reich.

Let's pause for a moment and reflect on what I am advocating you take upon yourself to do if you wish to avoid cancer.

To reiterate, as this is key to achieving a cancer resistant body environment and so very important on a daily basis, I recommend that you:

I. **Alkalize your body quickly by consistently eating the right foods and drinks full of Alkaline Minerals and Antioxidant Vitamins that lead to a slightly alkaline body state**

II. **Identify and eliminate all food that contains too much acidity from your diet.**

The chart below shows you **common acidic foods** that many of us consume every day without ever knowing the damage these foods inflict on our blood cells and tissues.

Partial List of foods to avoid because they contain TOO much ACIDITY:

Tomatoes	ACIDITY LEVEL: **4.30 - 4.90** Consumable when grown organically and completely ripe
Sweet peppers	ACIDITY LEVEL: **4.65 - 5.45**
Red beetroots	ACIDITY LEVEL: **5.30 - 6.60**
Sorrel	ACIDITY LEVEL: **4.5**

Oranges	**ACIDITY LEVEL:** **3.69 - 4.34**
Mandarins, tangerines	**ACIDITY LEVEL:** **3.32 - 4.48**
Grapefruits	**ACIDITY LEVEL:** **3.00 - 3.75**
Strawberries	**ACIDITY LEVEL:** **3.00 - 3.90** Consumable when grown organically and ripe
Raspberries	**ACIDITY LEVEL:** **3.22 - 3.95** Consumable when grown organically and ripe

Blackcurrant	**ACIDITY LEVEL:** **4.8 – 7.0** Consumable when grown organically and ripe
Redcurrant	**ACIDITY LEVEL:** **4.8 – 7.0** Consumable when grown organically and ripe
Gooseberries	**ACIDITY LEVEL:** **2.80 - 3.10**
Pineapples	**ACIDITY LEVEL:** **3.20 - 4.00**
Kiwis	**ACIDITY LEVEL:** **3.1 – 3.96**

Dates	**ACIDITY LEVEL:** **4.14 - 4.88**
Honey	**ACIDITY LEVEL:** **3.70 - 4.20** One teaspoon of honey a week is ok
Cocas, sodas	**ACIDITY LEVEL:** **2.0 – 4.0**
Champagne	**ACIDITY LEVEL:** **2.8 – 3.8**
White wines	**ACIDITY LEVEL:** **3.0 – 3.3**

Pink wines	**ACIDITY LEVEL:** **3.0 – 3.3**
Young red wines	**ACIDITY LEVEL:** **3.3 – 3.5**
Desserts	**ACIDITY LEVEL:** **1.6 – 3.0**
Candies	**ACIDITY LEVEL:** **1.6 – 3.0**
Vinegar	**ACIDITY LEVEL:** **2.40 - 3.40**

Pickles	ACIDITY LEVEL:
	5.10 - 5.40

The pH of soda drinks

Here is a chart of the acidity levels of some common Sodas:

SODA NAME	pH
Coke	ACIDITY LEVEL: 2.52
Diet Coke	ACIDITY LEVEL: 3.28

Coca Cola Zero	ACIDITY LEVEL: 3.28
Pepsi	ACIDITY LEVEL: 2.53
Diet Pepsi	ACIDITY LEVEL: 3.03
Dr. Pepper	ACIDITY LEVEL: 2.89

Diet Dr. Pepper	**ACIDITY LEVEL:** **3.16**
Cherry Coke	**ACIDITY LEVEL:** **2.52**
RC Cola	**ACIDITY LEVEL:** **2.38**
Mr. Pibb	**ACIDITY LEVEL:** **2.90**

Mountain Dew	ACIDITY LEVEL: 3.22
Diet Mountain Dew	ACIDITY LEVEL: 3.36
Sprite	ACIDITY LEVEL: 3.20
7 Up	ACIDITY LEVEL: 3.20

Diet 7 Up	ACIDITY LEVEL: **3.70**
Lemon Brisk	ACIDITY LEVEL: **2.86**
Lemon Nestea	ACIDITY LEVEL: **2.96**

Chapter 2

The Solution in detail

ALKALIZING and CANCER preventative MINERALS, ANTIOXIDANT VITAMINS and foods rich in them

As you can appreciate, there is a strong case to be argued that underpinning the ever increasing incidence of cancer in many countries, is the fact we humans throughout our lifetime unintentionally nourish our bodies with **very acidic foods** and **drinks** that are typical of the foods and beverages popular in most developed countries today.

It is perhaps surprising that many of the favorite beverages people drink are acid-forming: pasteurized juices which contain literally spoonfuls of sugar as well as the globally popular soda drinks which feature high acid pH rates in the case of Coke from 2.5 to 3.2 for Sprite as you no doubt noticed in the soda chart in Chapter 1. Aside from the acidic diet many people live their lives with, it is also a fact that **stress**, **anxiety**, and **fear** that we humans experience in our family and business lives also contribute quite measurably towards increased acidity levels in the body which creates the "perfect storm" incubator environment for cancer cell reproduction. Lack of alkalizing minerals and antioxidant vitamins in the body is a huge contributor to lots of illnesses including cancer. As a result the body's immune system becomes very weak and can't fight against disease. Two people will be exposed to the same bacteria and one of them will get sick, and the other one will stay perfectly healthy. Why? Because the immune system of the second person is very strong and killed the bacteria. Nowadays almost all of us are experiencing a lack to some degree, of the minerals and vitamins required by our system.

Given that everybody has cancer cells in their system it is useful to know how cancer cells produce the energy they need - which they do by using a fermentation process, which itself, **creates lactic acid**, further **increasing body acidity** and **reducing tissue oxygen levels**.

The significance of reduced levels of oxygen in body tissue was highlighted by Nobel Prize Laureate, Dr. Otto Warburg, who discovered that when he lowered the oxygen levels of tissues by 35 % for 48 hours, **normal cells** were found to be converted into **irreversible cancer cells**.

Fortunately, the positive effect of alkalizing minerals and antioxidant vitamins in destroying cancer cells is very well documented.

A. Keith Brewer, Ph.D. *"The high pH therapy for cancer tests on mice and humans".* PHARMACOL BIOCHEM BEHAV **21**: Suppl. 1, 1-5. 1984 stated:
"Mass spectrographic and isotope studies have shown that **potassium, rubidium,** *and especially* **cesium** *are most efficiently taken up by cancer cells. This uptake was*

*enhanced by **Vitamins A** and **C** as well as salts of **zinc** and **selenium**. The quantity of cesium taken up was sufficient to raise the cell to the 8 pH range where cancer cell mitosis (growth) ceases and the life of the cell is short".*

It is important that we spend sometime increasing our understanding about the different minerals that will contribute to an alkaline state for our body tissue and cells.

IMPORTANT ALKALIZING MINERALS FOR CANCER AVOIDANCE

Specifically, these are:
Potassium: **pH 14**
Cesium: **pH 14**
Calcium: **pH 12**
Magnesium: **pH 9**
Selenium: **pH 9**
Sodium: **pH 14**
Rubidium: **pH 14**

Selenium is a nutritional mineral that is critical to the body's defense against cancer and other illnesses involving **free radicals** and other **reactive oxygen species**.

Dr. Richard A. Passwater's research with selenium as a cancer preventative began in 1959, and over the decades, thousands of mechanistic studies, hundreds of animal studies, dozens of epidemiological (population) studies, and at least three published clinical supplementation trials have verified his findings.

On December 25, 1996, Dr. Larry Clark and his colleagues published their large, prospective, randomized, placebo-controlled, double-blind Nutritional Prevention of Cancer (NPC) clinical study in the Journal of the American Medical Association (JAMA 1996; 276:1957-1963). This landmark research effort showed that daily supplementation of diets with **200 micrograms of selenium** yeast cut the cancer death rate in half. That is cancer **mortality** was reduced 50 %. **Lung cancer** deaths were reduced 53%.

Total cancer incidence was reduced 37 % and the total carcinoma incidence was reduced 45%. In addition, the three leading sites of cancer had significantly lower **incidence**; **lung cancer** incidence was reduced 46 %, **prostate cancer** incidence was reduced 63 % and **colon cancer** incidence was reduced 58 %. There was a 17% reduction in all cause mortality, which when adjusted for sex, current smoking and age yielded a 21% reduction in deaths from all causes.

Throughout all of the mechanistic, animal and clinical studies of selenium it has been observed that not only is the incidence reduced, but also the severity and death rate have been even more greatly reduced suggesting that tumors are being destroyed, not just prevented. At the very least, the progression of cancer is delayed.

A large 2003 French study called SU.VI.MAX incorporated **100 micrograms of selenium** as selenomethione in its regimen that also included vitamins C and E, beta-carotene and zinc. It found that the supplements reduced cancer deaths by 37% and cancer incidence 30%.

Cesium, an extremely **alkaline mineral**, has been used effectively on cancer since the 1930s. Cesium chloride is considered a potent cancer treatment for even stage four levels of cancer and cancer metastasized throughout the body, including lymphoma and leukemia.

Calcium is a soft alkaline earth metal. Although none of the alkaline earths occur free in nature, calcium compounds are abundant. A lot of us will be surprised to find out that we can provide our bodies with plenty of calcium coming from vegetables, nuts, fruits, legumes, lentils, whole grains, etc.

For proper calcium absorption, you need to consume food sources that contain types of calcium that are easily digested, assimilated, and absorbed. It's important to know the special relationship between **magnesium** and **calcium**, as they rely on each other, and **both need** to be present for **proper absorption**. Usually it's in a 2:1 ratio, with two parts calcium to one part of magnesium. What would be interesting for you to know that **one cup of 1-percent low-fat milk** provides **305 mg of calcium** and **27 mg of magnesium.** You can calculate the rest…

As you can see because of the calcium-magnesium ratio in **dairy products**, our bodies **do not properly absorb** the **calcium** it contains. **Excess stores of calcium** accumulate in our **blood** and **urine** as a result can cause kidney problems, formation of kidney stones and gallstones unfortunately.

Magnesium is a crucial mineral that helps restore proper pH Balance. Magnesium is vital in assisting calcium and potassium uptake in addition to its alkalizing effect.

The role of magnesium in cancer is quickly gaining interest

among researchers because of recent studies showing protective effects against multiple cancers. The most recent studies from Netherlands on colon cancer have shown that every additional 100 mg of magnesium daily may reduce the risk of colorectal cancer by 12 %. The EPIC Cohort study from Europe showed that every 100 mg/day increase in dietary magnesium reduced the risk of pancreatic cancer by 21 %.

Magnesium plays a major role as a cancer preventative by taking part as a co-factor in over 300 enzyme systems and is found in every tissue of the human body.

Magnesium plays a critical function in DNA repair, cell differentiation, angiogenesis and proliferation. All this is relevant for cancer. Magnesium deficiency has also been linked directly to oxidative stress and inflammation, and now, to **increased cancer risk**.

Statistics show that 79% of American adults don't get enough magnesium in their diets. The current recommended daily (or dietary) allowance is 320 mg/day for women and 420 mg/day for men.

Potassium is an alkalizing mineral that the body needs to work normally. It helps move nutrients into cells and waste products out of cells. Potassium helps regulate major body functions, including normal heart rhythm, blood pressure, water balance in the body, digestion, nerve impulses, muscle contractions, and pH balance.

Now let us take a look at ANTIOXIDANT VITAMINS WHICH ARE IMPORTANT FOR A CANCER AVOIDANCE DIET

Specifically, these are:

Vitamin A and the Carotenoids

Vitamin A carotenoids are naturally occurring in fruits and vegetables which are yellow, red and green in color. This antioxidant family includes alpha-carotene, beta-carotene, lycopene, lutein and zeaxanthin. Working effectively as **anti-cancer agents**, carotenoids decrease the risk of cataracts and age-related macular degeneration as well as helping to inhibit **heart disease**. The body converts carotenoid energy into vitamin A and reduces the oxidation of DNA.

Vitamin C

Vitamin C works in conjunction with vitamin E to maintain its potency. Due to its water solubility, vitamin C works in bodily fluids as an effective free-radical scavenger. According to the book "Prescription for Nutritional Healing" by Dr. Phyllis A. Balch, the **cells** of the **brain** and **spinal cord** can be protected by significant amounts of natural **vitamin C**. This powerful antioxidant also guards against atherosclerosis by preventing free radical damage to the artery walls.

I would like you to pay attention to the difference between Natural Vitamins vs. Synthetic.

Natural vs. Synthetic.

We will start with Vitamin C as most sources equate vitamin C with ascorbic acid, and many people think they are the same thing. Actually they are not. **Ascorbic acid** is a distillate of naturally occurring vitamin C. In addition to ascorbic acid, **vitamin C must include** rutin, bioflavonoids, Factor K, Factor J, Factor P, Tyrosinase, Ascorbinogen, and other components.

In addition, mineral co-factors must be available in proper amounts.

"If any of these parts are missing, there is no vitamin C, no vitamin C activity. When some of them are present, the body will draw on its own stores to make up the differences, so that the whole vitamin may be present. Only then will vitamin activity take place, provided that all other conditions and co-factors are present. Ascorbic acid is described merely as the "antioxidant wrapper" portion of vitamin C; **ascorbic acid protects** the **functional parts** of the **vitamin C** from **rapid oxidation** or **breakdown**." (p. 58 "Vitamin C: A Lesson in Keeping An Open Mind" The Nutrition Report)

It is useful to note that Vitamins are not individual molecular compounds. Vitamins are biological complexes. They are multi-step biochemical interactions whose action is dependent upon a number of variables within the biological terrain. Vitamin activity only takes place when all conditions are met within that environment, and when all co-factors and components of the entire vitamin complex are present and working together. Effective Vitamin activity is even more than the sum of all those parts; it also involves timing.

Vitamins cannot be isolated from their complexes and still perform their specific life functions within the cells. When isolated into artificial commercial forms, like ascorbic acid, these purified synthetics act as drugs in the body.

Mother Nature knew what she was doing when she created vitamin C-rich fruits, berries and plants. Scientists now know that vitamin C isolates such as ascorbic acid do not provide the health benefits that whole food forms of vitamin C do.

Vitamin E

Useful for preventing the oxidation of fats, vitamin E prevents the cell's protective coatings from becoming rancid due to the **oxidation** of **free radicals**. Vitamin E is fat-soluble. It enhances the **immune response**, helps prevent cataracts and decreases the risk for coronary artery disease. In order for the body to maintain adequate levels of vitamin E, the antioxidant zinc must also be present.

Alpha-tocopherol is the most biologically active form of vitamin E, and its **natural form** consists of **one isomer.** In contrast, **synthetic alpha-tocopherol** contains **eight different isomers**, of which only one (about 12 percent of the synthetic molecule) is identical to natural vitamin E. The other seven isomers range in potency from 21 percent to 90 percent of natural d-alpha-tocopherol.

This may appear to be arcane nutritional chemistry, but I include it as it is key to understanding how the body absorbs **natural** and **synthetic** supplements differently. Molecular structure determines how the body uses vitamin E.

Researchers have found that natural vitamin E assimilates into the body far better than synthetic versions. Specific binding and transport proteins produced in the liver select the natural **d-alpha form of vitamin E** and largely ignore all other forms.

On a supplement label, **natural vitamin E** is listed as **d-alpha tocopherol, d-alpha tocopheryl acetate,** or **d-alpha tocopheryl succinate**. In contrast, **synthetic forms** of vitamin E are labeled with a **dl- prefix**.

Biochemically speaking, vitamin E can be either right or left handed. This is indicated with the letters D and L. The form that exists in our food and the form that our bodies need is the D form: D-alpha tocopherol. **The L form does not work in our bodies.**

Synthetic vitamin E is not the same as natural vitamin E and has lower biological activity. When vitamin E is made synthetically a mixture of the D and L forms is automatically produced and cannot be separated. This is called DL-alpha tocopherol and, although much less expensive than natural D-alpha tocopherol, is not biologically active. In fact, **recent scientific studies** have indicated that synthetic vitamin E **does not stay** in the body nearly as long as natural vitamin E, making it a **much less effective protector**.

According to new research on the subject, **avocados** are now recognized as the richest *fruit* source of vitamin E, closely followed by nectarines, grapes, and then peaches. Avocados are also the best fruit source of **lutein**, the compound that protects against **cataract formation** and **macular degeneration**. (Nut Week 01:31(24):7)

The National Academy of Sciences recognized natural vitamin E as the standard by which to judge synthetics. Natural vitamin E contains the molecule humans assimilate most effectively.

Coenzyme Q10

Though coenzyme Q10 is not technically a vitamin, it is produced naturally in the body and levels often decrease with age. Found in highest concentrations in the heart and liver, coenzyme Q10 plays a crucial role in the **generation** of proper **cellular energy.** Working in the **mitochondria** of the cell, coenzyme Q10 helps to metabolize carbohydrates and fats and has a natural anti-aging effect. Supplementing the diet with coenzyme Q10 may be especially beneficial for heart patients, as it is known to increase circulation and stimulate the **immune system.**

Alpha-Lipoic Acid

Alpha-Lipoic Acid is working as a "recycler" of vitamins C and E, and restores the antioxidant properties of vitamins after they have **neutralized free radicals** in the body. Stimulating the absorption of other vitamins, alpha-lipoic acid is especially beneficial for **detoxifying the liver** of metal pollutants as well as lowering blood cholesterol levels.

Our body digests and benefits most from minerals and vitamins when they are taken into the body as substances within **wholesome foods** like the organic **vegetables, fruits, whole grains, legumes, wild fish, organic eggs** and other foods you will become familiar with from the charts contained in this book.

First, before we come to the chart below I would like to focus you to take a close look at an often overlooked **extraordinary green vegetable** and the studies and findings in relation to its cancer preventative qualities.

You'll find nearly 100 studies in PubMed (the health research database at the National Library of Medicine in Washington, D.C.) that are focused on **Brussels sprouts**, and over half of those studies involve the significant health benefits of this cruciferous vegetable in **relation to cancer**. This connection between **Brussels sprouts** and **cancer prevention** exists since Brussels sprouts provide special nutrient support for three body systems that are closely connected with **cancer development** as well as **cancer prevention**.

These three systems are:

1. The body's detox system
2. Its inflammatory/anti-inflammatory system.
3. Its antioxidant system

Chronic imbalances in any of these three systems can increase risk of cancer, and when imbalances in all three systems occur simultaneously, the **risk of cancer** increases significantly. Among **all types of cancer**, prevention of the following cancer types is most closely associated with intake of Brussels sprouts: **bladder cancer, breast cancer, colon cancer, lung cancer, prostate cancer, and ovarian cancer.**

Research has shown that the cancer protection we get from Brussels sprouts is largely related to four specific cancer-preventive components in special combination found in this cruciferous vegetable.

A recent study has shown improved stability of DNA inside of our **white blood cells** after daily consumption of **Brussels sprouts in the amount of 1.25 cups**. Interestingly, it's the ability of certain compounds in Brussels sprouts to block the activity of sulphotransferase enzymes that researchers believe to be responsible for these DNA-protective benefits.

Brussels sprouts are now known to top the list of commonly eaten cruciferous vegetables in terms of health benefit. Their total glucosinolate content has been shown to be greater than the amount found in mustard greens, turnip greens, cabbage, kale, cauliflower, or broccoli. **Glucosinolates** are important **phytonutrients** for our health because they are the chemical starting points for a variety of **cancer-protective substances**. All cruciferous vegetables contain glucosinolates and have great health benefits for this reason. But it's recent research that's made us realize how especially **valuable** Brussels sprouts are in this regard.

Brussels sprouts have been used to determine the potential impact of cruciferous vegetables on thyroid function. In a recent study, 5 ounces of Brussels sprouts were consumed on a daily basis for 4 consecutive weeks by a small group of healthy adults and were not found to have an unwanted impact on their thyroid function. This study puts at least one large stamp of approval on Brussels sprouts as a food that can provide fantastic health benefits without putting the thyroid gland at risk.

If you have not previously been very fond of this vegetable because of its taste or smell, I am happy to show you that you can cook them in several very delicious ways:

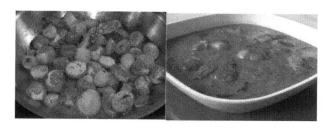

Brussels Sprouts and Detox Support

The detox support provided by Brussels sprouts is quite extensive. *First*, there is evidence from human studies that **enzyme systems in our cells** required for **detoxification** of **cancer-causing substances** can be activated by compounds made from **glucosinolates** found in Brussels sprouts.

Second, the body's detox system **requires** ample supplies of **sulphur** to work effectively, and Brussels sprouts are **rich** in sulphur-containing nutrients. Sulphur is connected with both the **smell** and **taste** of Brussels sprouts, and too much sulphur aroma is often associated with overcooking of this vegetable. Sulphur-containing nutrients help support what is commonly referred to as Phase 2 of detoxification. *Third*, our body's **detox system** needs strong **antioxidant support** - especially during what is called Phase 1 of detoxification. Brussels sprouts are able to provide that kind of support because they are an excellent source of **vitamin C**, a very good source of **beta-carotene** and **manganese**, and a good source of **vitamin E**. Brussels sprouts also contain a wide variety of antioxidant phytonutrients, including many antioxidant flavonoids. Finally, there is evidence that the DNA in our cells is protected by naturally occurring substances in Brussels sprouts, and since many environmental toxins can trigger unwanted change in our DNA, Brussels sprouts can help prevent these toxin-triggered DNA changes.

Brussels Sprouts and Inflammatory/Anti-inflammatory Support

Chronic unwanted inflammation is also a risk factor for **many types of cancer**. Exposure to **environmental toxins**, chronic overuse of prescription or **over-the-counter medications**, chronic excessive stress, chronic lack of exercise, chronic lack of sleep, and a **low quality diet** can all contribute to our risk of **unwanted inflammation**.

Brussels sprouts and lots of other green vegetables and fruits can help us avoid chronic, excessive inflammation through a variety of nutrient benefits.

Glucosinolates found in Brussels sprouts help to regulate the body's **inflammatory/anti-inflammatory system** and prevent unwanted inflammation.

A second important anti-inflammatory nutrient found in Brussels sprouts is **vitamin K**. Vitamin K is a direct regulator of inflammatory responses, and we need optimal intake of this vitamin in order to avoid chronic, excessive inflammation.

Just for you to compare: the amount of **Vitamin K** in organic **Brussels sprouts** is **218.9** mcg and in organic **carrots** is **10.7** mcg.

A third important anti-inflammatory component in Brussels sprouts is not one that you might expect. It's their **omega-3** fatty acids. We don't tend to think about vegetables in general as **important sources** of omega-3s, and certainly no vegetables that are as low in total fat as Brussels sprouts. But 100 calories' worth of Brussels sprouts (about 1.5 cups) provide about **430 milligrams** of the most basic omega-3 fatty acid (called alpha-linolenic acid, or ALA). That amount is more than one-third of the daily ALA amount recommended by the **National Academy of Sciences** in the Dietary Reference Intake recommendations, and it's about half of the ALA contained in one teaspoon of whole flaxseeds. Omega-3 fatty acids are the building blocks for the one of the body's most effective families of anti-inflammatory messaging molecules.

Brussels Sprouts and Antioxidant Support

As mentioned earlier, Brussels sprouts are an important dietary source of many **vitamin antioxidants**, including vitamins C, E, and A (in the form of beta-carotene) as well as the **alkaline minerals** such as **potassium, calcium magnesium, selenium** etc. Flavonoid antioxidants like isorhamnetin, quercitin, and kaempferol are also found in Brussels sprouts, as are the antioxidants **caffeic acid** and **ferulic acid**. In fact, one study examining total intake of antioxidant polyphenols in France found Brussels sprouts to be a more important dietary contributor to these antioxidants than any other cruciferous vegetable, including broccoli. Some of the antioxidant compounds found in Brussels sprouts may be somewhat rare in foods overall.

Treated as a group, the antioxidant nutrients described

above provide support not only for Phase 1 of the body's detoxification process but also for all of the body's cells that are at risk of oxidative damage from overly reactive oxygen-containing molecules. **Chronic oxidative stress**— meaning chronic presence of overly reactive oxygen-containing molecules and cumulative damage to tissue by these molecules — is a risk factor for the development of **most cancer types**.

More about INFLAMATION

Inflammation is a huge topic these days as recent research indicates that there is no longer any doubt that inflammation produces a cascade of events responsible for most chronic diseases including cancer. Often medical doctors prescribe drug treatment and there are times that this is what is needed. There are also instances when alternatives are appropriate and I would like you to be well equipped with information about herbs and vegetables that have **anti-inflammatory properties**. Some of them are widely available and you can include them in your diet as preventative as well as enjoying their delicious taste. Many herbs can work on inflammation in a multi-faceted holistic and balanced way and you don't get the side effects like from drugs.

Anti-INFLAMATORY Herbs and Vegetables:

Turmeric (*Curcuma longa*) 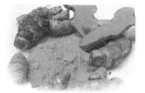	Over the past several years, numerous studies have emerged on the benefits of Turmeric and on its anti-cancerous properties. Curcumin, which is present in Turmeric (Curcuma Longa), is a powerful antioxidant. Turmeric is also a powerful anti-inflammatory and is very effective in treating all kinds of inflammatory diseases as well as arthritis, tendinitis, injuries, etc. The plant is also a powerful blood purifier and is highly effective in reducing excessive cholesterol. Turmeric is very safe and has been used in Chinese medicine for more than 4,000 years.
Ginger: (Zingiber officinalis) 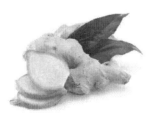	Ginger has a long history of use as an anti-inflammatory and many of its constituents have been identified as having anti-inflammatory properties. Ginger has been shown to be more effective against bacterial staph infections than antibiotics. It can kill cancer cells. Its anti-inflammatory effects are

	already famous. It can resolve brain inflammations and ease or cure a variety of gut problems, such as ulcerative colitis and acid reflux. And ginger can even alleviate the effects of gamma radiation. It has also been indicated for arthritis, fevers, headaches, toothaches, coughs, bronchitis, osteoarthritis, rheumatoid arthritis, to ease tendonitis, lower cholesterol and blood pressure and aid in preventing internal blood clots.
Garlic 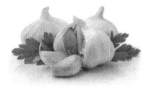	Medical scientists, who have new evidence of its potency against cancer and heart disease, are now rediscovering garlic, recognized for its healing powers in ancient times. Sulphides, which are found in garlic in large amounts, stop the growth of tumors and inhibit carcinogens. According to the National Cancer Institute, garlic lies among the top of the list of foods ingested as a potential weapon against many types of cancer. Garlic is a natural, potent antibiotic, antiviral and antifungal herb. A study done at Boston

	University School of Medicine conducted tests in which garlic proved to be as effective as an antibiotic in killing 14 types of bacteria in reoccurring infections. Garlic has also been shown in some studies to decrease high blood sugar, boost metabolism, inhibit growth and formation of cancer cells, prevent inflammation, and alleviate allergies and asthma.
Cardamom 	The study, published in the April-June 2005 issue of "Asian Pacific Journal of Cancer Prevention," found cancer cell reproduction was diminished and apoptosis -- programmed cell death -- was increased in response to supplementation with three doses of 0.5 percent cardamom extract per day for eight weeks. Additionally, cardamom had anti-inflammatory effects, as observed by the inhibition of cyclooxygenase 2, also known as COX2 -- a pro-inflammatory enzyme.
Cayenne	Cayenne pepper has anti-inflammatory, antioxidant, antiseptic, diuretic, analgesic,

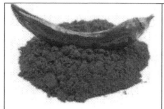

expectorant, and diaphoretic properties. According to an article published in the "Indian Journal of Cancer" in Jan-March 2010, there are other substance in chili peppers and cayenne, known collectively as capsaicinoids, offer anticancer benefits. Capsaicin appears to induce cancer cell death by blocking several proteins and interrupting signaling pathways required for cancer cell growth survival and proliferation.

Chives

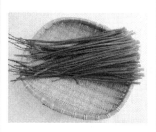

Chives help inhibit the growth of tumors and cancer. The small onions have been found helpful in the treatment of esophageal, stomach, prostrate and gastrointestinal tract cancers. Selenium in the small onion helps to protect cells from the effects of toxins and free radicals. Like most plants in the allium group, chives have antibiotic properties. The natural antibacterial and antiviral agents in the vegetable work with vitamin C to destroy harmful microbes. This makes the

	plant an excellent natural defense against the common cold, flu and certain yeast infections.
Nutmeg 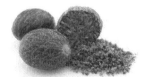	Nutmeg which is made by grinding the seeds produced by the nutmeg tree offers help for those fighting cancer battles with certain forms of leukemia. A recent medical study has shown that nutmeg extract causes cancer cells to self-destruct in leukemia patients. Nutmeg is known to have anti-inflammatory properties and can be used to treat joint and muscle pain.
Cilantro 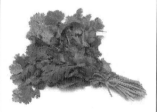	Cilantro or, more commonly, coriander is a potent herb that has anti-cancer properties. The prevalent anti-oxidants in cilantro are beta-carotene, quercetin and rutin. This herb, normally used in chelation therapy for people suffering from lead poisoning, helps remove free radicals by getting rid of the heavy metals in your body. Dr. Yoshiaki Omura from the Heart Disease Research Foundation, New York, NY, USA, has actually found that fresh cilantro removes heavy metals –

	and with it the free radicals too – from the body in less than 2 weeks.
Cinnamon	Cinnamon is a common and flavorful spice that contains polyphenols. The polyphenol compounds help reduce cancer risk by preventing damage to healthy cells. Cinnamon, which is made from the dried tree bark of Asian cinnamon trees, has also shown evidence of having the ability to stop the cancer cell growth of melanoma.
Cloves	Cloves is a common spice often used around Thanksgiving and Christmas for adding flavor to Holiday dinner recipes, and the same spice that flavors your Christmas ham will also reduce your cancer risk by protecting your skin cells from malignant melanomas.
Black Pepper	Angiogenesis is a physiological process enabling the growth of new blood vessels from pre-existing ones. A vital mechanism for wound healing, angiogenesis is also a key process involved in tumor growth and progression. Several

	previous studies suggest that piperine, an alkaloid compound found abundantly in black pepper, has diverse physiological actions including the ability to kill cancer cells.
Basil	Basil is well known for its medicinal value. Apart from having anti-inflammatory, blood pressure lowering, and nervous system stimulating properties, this popular herb has been found to have chemo-protective potential for colon cancer. In fact, a study found that basil played a significant role in reducing colon tumors in experimental animals. In cell culture and animal studies basil has been found to exhibit antimicrobial, anti-inflammatory, anti-diabetic, antioxidant and anti-cancer activity.
Parsley	Parsley is rich in antioxidants like vitamin C, beta-carotene and quercetin, but also contains less well known flavonoids like apigenin, luteolin and chrysoeroil. Apigenin research studies have associated it with a

	decreased risk of pancreatic cancer, leukemia, cervical and ovarian cancer. Apigenin has also been shown to interfere with cancer cell proliferation, exhibiting strong anti-tumor properties. Not only does apigenin possesses remarkable anti-cancer properties, it's also a powerful anti-inflammatory and antioxidant. Chrysoeroil has also been studied for its potential anti-cancer benefits, particularly with regards to preventing breast cancer.
Chamomile 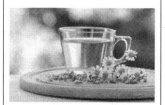	Recent and on-going research has identified chamomile's specific anti-inflammatory, anti-bacterial, anti-allergenic and sedative properties, validating its long-held reputation. Most evaluations of tumor growth inhibition by chamomile involve studies with apigenin, which is one of the bioactive constituents of chamomile. Studies on preclinical models of skin, prostate, breast and ovarian cancer have shown promising growth inhibitory effects.
Rosemary	Rosmarinic acid, a natural polyphenolic

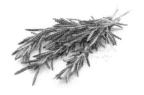

antioxidant found in rosemary, has been found to have anti-bacterial, anti-inflammatory, and anti-oxidant functions. Rosemary contains proven anti-inflammatory properties that can reduce the risk of colon cancer.

Stinging Nettle

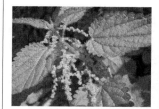

In ancient Greek times, the stinging nettle was used mainly as a diuretic and laxative. Now the plant is used for many cures; illnesses include **cancer** and **diabetes**.
Stinging Nettle has **anti-inflammatory properties** and treats illness of the urinary track.
The stinging nettle is a **blood purifier** and thus cleans eczema internally. It is the best blood purifier available and has an influence over the pancreas. Stinging nettle also assists in **lowering blood sugar**. Nettle has been studied extensively and has shown promise in treating Alzheimer's disease, arthritis, asthma, bladder infections, bronchitis, bursitis, gingivitis, gout, hives, kidney stones, laryngitis, multiple sclerosis, PMS, prostate enlargement, sciatica, and tendinitis!

The best, as you know, is to have everything in moderation. Sometimes people find out for example what a good healing power garlic has and start consuming it every day, which is quite dangerous. As well as having healing power, like everything else it can become a poison when taken in high doses. When you nourish your precious body with a variety of different fruits, vegetables, good carbs and good fat then your cells have plenty of good quality building material to operate and regenerate with. It will not take long for you to see the difference in your health!

One of the very important parts of our body, which is our brain, consists of about 100 billion brain cells called **neurons** that drive our thinking, learning, feeling and states of being. To do their best work, neurons need good fats, protein, complex carbohydrates, micronutrients - vitamins, minerals and phytonutrients - and water. Your quality of thinking depends dramatically on the quality of food you provide for your brain.

Good quality food provides proper function for our brain as about one-fifth of the oxygen, nutrients and energy consumed by a person go directly to the brain, which is primarily composed of fat and water.

Proper nutrition enhances neurogenesis, the process of generating new brain cells.

Your brain cells need two times more energy than the other cells in your body.

Neurons are communicating with each other and have a high demand for energy because they're always in a state of metabolic activity. Even during your sleep, neurons are still at work repairing and rebuilding their worn out structural components.

They are manufacturing enzymes and neurotransmitters that must be transported out to the very ends of their– nerve branches, some that can be several inches, or feet, away.

It would be useful for you as well to understand the difference between high-glycemic-index foods, which is mainly processed carbohydrates like everything made from white flower, white rice, white sugar, etc. All this processed food spikes the level of your blood sugar quite dramatically, which can lead to diabetes, heart disease, cancer, obesity, etc.

Diets rich in high-glycemic-index foods, have been linked to an increased risk for diabetes, heart disease and overweight and there is preliminary work linking high-glycemic diets to age-related macular degeneration, ovulatory infertility and colorectal cancer.

One of the most important factors that determine a food's glycemic index is how much it has been processed. Milling and grinding **removes** the **fiber-rich outer bran** and the **vitamin- and mineral-rich inner germ**, leaving mostly the starchy endosperm.

Eating **whole grains, beans, legumes, fruits and vegetables**—all foods with a **low glycemic index**—is indisputably good for many aspects of health as well as very important food for your brain. The quality of your thinking, the level of your energy, the strength of your immune system and the shape of your body depends very much on the quality of the food you are providing for it! You will be very excited and quite surprised to see how all unwanted fat will be gently melting as soon as you provide your body with good fats, good carbs, plenty of vegetables, legumes and fruits.

The choice is YOURS as it is your body and you are the only One who chooses what to feed it with! You can treat it to what it wants or not!

Talking about keeping your healthy food delicious and having a good variety I thought you might like to explore one or two of these recipes into your new diet:

Delicious recipe for Brussels Sprouts Curry with Pumpkin and Pomegranate

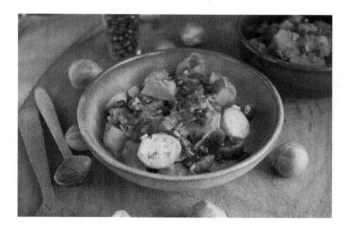

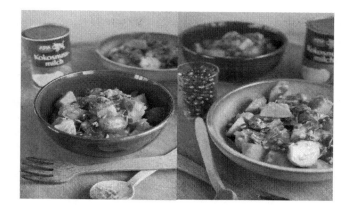

As I promise you, health sustaining food can always be delicious and here below is a one example of it as a quick and very easy vegetable curry made with Brussels sprouts and pumpkin. It is flavorful and delicious served with some warm homemade wholegrain bread or brown, black rice:

30 g Ginger
1 Onion
1 clove Garlic
350 g Brussels sprout
350 g Pumpkin
1 tbsp Olive oil
2 tsp Curry powder
200 ml Coconut milk
200 ml Vegetable stock
Sea salt according to your taste
1-2 tsp Lime juice
2 tbsp Cilantro or parsley, chopped
Some pomegranate seeds

- Finely dice the ginger, onion, and garlic. Rinse the Brussels sprouts and remove any wilted outer leaves.

Trim the woody bottoms and cut in half. Cut the pumpkin into inch pieces.

- Heat olive oil in a pan together with diced ginger, onion and garlic. Cook until aromatic, about 2 minutes. Add in Brussels sprouts and pumpkin. Cook for 5 minutes. Sprinkle the curry powder over and stir until well blended.

Pour in coconut milk and vegetable stock. Bring to a boil and cook, covered, over medium-heat for 15 minutes. Season with sea salt and lime juice. Garnish with cilantro leaves and pomegranate seeds.

Now, here is a vegetable, by the name of Mung Bean Sprouts, that most people have never come across that is worth mentioning too.

Mung Bean Sprouts Salad with Parsley Root and Carrot

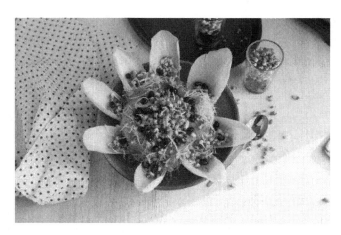

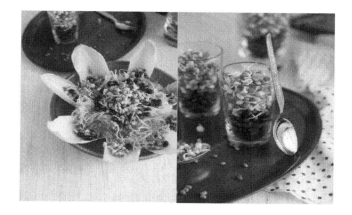

Mung bean sprouts contain various vitamins, in addition to an assortment of minerals including **calcium, iron, and potassium.** They are free of cholesterol, and are ideal for anyone counting calories. Bean sprouts are gaining popularity as a health food, appearing in a wide variety of dishes from salads to soups, wraps or just as a healthy snack. Making sprouts at home is easier than you think and they are generally fresher and better than any store bought one.

100 g Mung bean sprouts
100 g Parsley root, finely grated
50 g Carrot, finely grated
8 Belgian endive leaves
1 tbsp Pomegranate seeds
Lemon Juice
Olive oil
Sea Salt and pepper

- Peel and finely grate parsley root and carrot with a mandolin. Arrange Belgian endive leaves in a salad bowl. Place the grated vegetables in the center. Scatter the mung bean sprouts and pomegranate seeds over.

•

Add the olive oil, lemon juice and sea salt and pepper to taste and toss gently the grated vegetables, mung bean sprouts and pomegranate seeds together.

Garlic Mushrooms

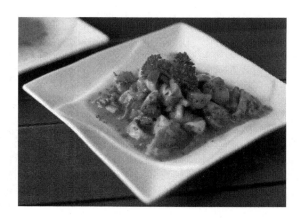

Ingredients:

60 ml Extra virgin olive oil
500 g Mushrooms, thinly sliced
3 clove Garlic, minced
60 ml Dry sherry
1 tbsp Fresh lemon juice
Pinch of dried chili flakes
Sea salt and pepper to taste
1 tbsp Parsley, chopped

Method:

Heat a skillet over medium-high heat. Pour in olive oil and
swirl to coat the bottom. Add in sliced mushrooms and
minced garlic. Cook, stirring frequently, for about 2
minutes.

Reduce the heat to medium. Drizzle in the sherry and
lemon juice. Season with chili flakes, salt and pepper.
Stir to combine. Cook until the mushrooms are
softened. Stir in chopped parsley. Stir to combine and
dish off.

To give you more ideas how your vegetables can be
consumed in a quite delicious way let me share with you the
idea of cooking with the many vegetables that you enjoy a
variety of different curried dishes:

Vegetable Curry dishes:

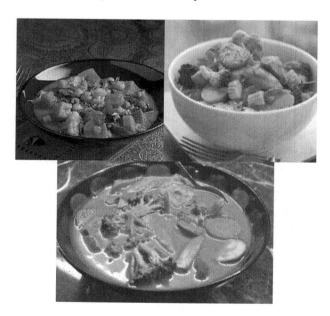

Generally speaking you can use any vegetables according to your own taste (apart from the ones which are very acidic of course) and have them cooked with delicious coconut milk and good quality curry powder or curry paste. Usually curry powder ingredients are very healthy including Cumin, Coriander seed, Garlic, Fenugreek, Ginger, Turmeric, Cayenne Paper, Chili, etc. In the chart above you learned about the anti-inflammatory properties of these ingredients.

The benefits of coconut milk are very well known too. Coconut milk helps control weight and keeps blood sugar level under a check. Also, it helps you feel full faster and hence very beneficial for people who are trying to lose weight. If you feel full, you tend to eat less. Moreover, it also reduces your **bad cholesterol** and is a great cure for **arthritis** and **joint pains**. Coconut milk has some beauty benefits too. It **moisturizes** your skin and nourishes it from within making it look beautiful and soft, I think Ladies will find this part beneficial too.

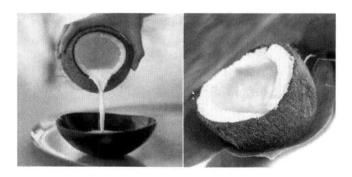

More coconut milk benefits:

Decreases the risk of joint inflammation:
Selenium is an important antioxidant. It controls the free

radicals and thereby helps in relieving the symptoms of arthritis. It is observed that people with low levels of selenium may suffer from rheumatoid arthritis.

Helps in lowering high blood pressure:
People who are concerned about their blood pressure will not face any problem consuming foods containing potassium. Potassium helps in lowering blood pressure levels in the body.

Helps in maintaining healthy immune system:
Coconut milk helps in warding off colds and coughs by keeping the immune system healthy. It supplies vitamin C to the body which boosts the immune system.

Promotes the health of prostate gland:
Zinc plays a vital role in promoting the health of prostate gland. A preliminary study showed that it slows down the activities of cancer cells.

Now let's take a more detailed look at the key alkalizing minerals and antioxidant vitamins that help your body achieve its natural level of alkalinity and which are contained in widely available vegetables:

Best Alkalizing Vegetables with Mineral and Vitamin content details

Vegetable	Amount	Minerals Contained	Vitamins Contained
Alfalfa, sprouted	One cup of raw, sprouted alfalfa seeds contains 1.32 grams of protein, 8 calories and 0.6 grams of dietary fiber.	Potassium - 26 mg Phosphorus - 23 mg Magnesium - 9 mg Calcium - 11 mg Iron - 0.32 mg Sodium - 2 mg Zinc - 0.3 mg Copper - 0.052 mg Manganese - 0.062 mg Selenium - 0.2 mcg Also contains small amounts of other minerals.	Vitamin C - 2.7 mg Vitamin B1 (thiamine) - 0.025 mg Vitamin B2 (riboflavin) - 0.042 mg Niacin - 0.159 mg Pantothenic Acid - 0.186 mg Vitamin B6 - 0.011 mg Folate - 12 mcg Vitamin A - 51 IU Vitamin K - 10.1 mcg Vitamin E - 0.01 mg Contains some other vitamins in small amounts.
Amaranth leaves	One cup of amaranth leaves, cooked, boiled, drained with no added salt has 2.79 grams protein and 28 calories.	Potassium - 846 mg Phosphorus - 95 mg Magnesium - 73 mg Calcium - 276 mg Iron - 2.98 mg Zinc - 1.16 mg Manganese - 1.137 mg Sodium - 28 mg Copper - 0.209 mg Selenium - 1.2 mcg Also contains small amounts of other minerals.	Vitamin C - 54.3 mg Vitamin B1 (thiamine) - 0.026 mg Vitamin B2 (riboflavin) - 0.177 mg Niacin - 0.738 mg Pantothenic Acid - 0.082 mg Vitamin B6 - 0.234 mg Folate - 75 mcg Vitamin A - 3656 IU Contains some other vitamins in small amounts.
Artichoke	One medium artichoke cooked with no added salt has 3.47 grams protein, 64 calories and	Potassium - 343 mg Phosphorus - 88 mg Magnesium - 50 mg Calcium - 25 mg Iron - 0.73 mg	Vitamin C - 8.9 mg Niacin - 1.332 mg Vitamin B1 (thiamine) - 0.06 mg Vitamin B2 (riboflavin) - 0.107 mg

	10.3 grams of fiber.	Zinc - 0.48 mg Copper - 0.152 mg Manganese - 0.27 mg Selenium - 0.2 mcg Sodium - 72 mg Also contains small amounts of other minerals.	Vitamin B6 - 0.097 mg Pantothenic Acid - 0.288 mg Folate - 107 mcg Vitamin A - 16 IU Vitamin K - 17.8 mcg Vitamin E - 0.23 mg Contains some other vitamins in small amounts.
Asparagus	Half cup (about 6 spears) cooked with no added salt contains 2.16 grams of protein, 20 calories and 1.8 grams of fiber.	Potassium - 202 mg Phosphorus - 49 mg Calcium - 21 mg Iron - 0.82 mg Sodium - 13 mg Magnesium - 13 mg Zinc - 0.54 mg Copper - 0.149 mg Manganese - 0.139 mg Selenium - 5.5 mcg Also contains small amounts of other minerals.	Vitamin A - 905 IU Vitamin C - 6.9 mg Niacin - 0.976 mg Vitamin B1 (thiamine) - 0.146 mg Vitamin B2 (riboflavin) - 0.125 mg Pantothenic Acid - 0.203 mg Vitamin B6 - 0.071 mg Folate - 134 mcg Vitamin K - 45.5 mcg Vitamin E - 1.35 mg Contains some other vitamins in small amounts.
Bamboo shoots	One cup of bamboo shoots, cooked, boiled, drained with no added salt has 1.84 grams protein, 14 calories and 1.2 grams dietary fiber.	Potassium - 640 mg Phosphorus - 24 mg Magnesium - 4 mg Calcium - 14 mg Iron - 0.29 mg Sodium - 5 mg Zinc - 0.56 mg Copper - 0.098 mg Manganese - 0.136 mg Selenium - 0.5 mcg Also contains small amounts of other minerals.	Niacin - 0.36 mg Vitamin B1 (thiamine) - 0.024 mg Vitamin B2 (riboflavin) - 0.06 mg Pantothenic Acid - 0.079 mg Vitamin B6 - 0.118 mg Folate - 2 mcg Contains some other vitamins in small amounts.
Bok Choy	One cup of Bok Choy (Pak Choi),	Potassium - 631 mg Phosphorus - 49	Vitamin C - 44.2 mg Niacin - 0.728 mg

	cooked, boiled, drained with no added salt has 2.65 grams protein, 20 calories and 1.7 grams dietary fiber.	mg Magnesium - 19 mg Calcium - 158 mg Iron - 1.77 mg Zinc - 0.29 mg Copper - 0.032 mg Manganese - 0.245 mg Selenium - 0.7 mcg Sodium - 58 mg Also contains small amounts of other minerals.	Vitamin B1 (thiamine) - 0.054 mg Vitamin B2 (riboflavin) - 0.107 mg Pantothenic Acid - 0.134 mg Vitamin B6 - 0.282 mg Folate - 70 mcg Vitamin A - 7223 IU Vitamin E - 0.15 mg Vitamin K - 57.8 mcg Contains some other vitamins in small amounts.
Broccoli	Half cup of broccoli, cooked with no added salt contains 1.86 grams protein, 27 calories and 2.6 grams dietary fiber.	Potassium - 229 mg Phosphorus - 52 mg Calcium - 31 mg Sodium - 32 mg Magnesium - 16 mg Iron - 0.52 mg Zinc - 0.35 mg Copper - 0.048 mg Manganese - 0.151 mg Selenium - 1.2 mcg Also contains small amounts of other minerals.	Vitamin A - 1207 IU Vitamin C - 50.6 mg Niacin - 0.431 mg Vitamin B1 (thiamine) - 0.049 mg Vitamin B2 (riboflavin) - 0.096 mg Vitamin B6 - 0.156 mg Pantothenic Acid - 0.48 mg Folate - 84 mcg Vitamin K - 110 mcg Vitamin E - 1.13 mg Contains some other vitamins in small amounts.
Brussels Sprouts	One cup of Brussels Sprouts, cooked, boiled, drained with no added salt has 3.98 grams protein, 56 calories and 4.1 grams dietary fiber.	Potassium - 495 mg Phosphorus - 87 mg Magnesium - 31 mg Calcium - 56 mg Iron - 1.87 mg Zinc - 0.51 mg Copper - 0.129 mg Manganese - 0.354 mg Selenium - 2.3 mcg Sodium - 33 mg	Vitamin C - 96.7 mg Niacin - 0.947 mg Vitamin B1 (thiamine) - 0.167 mg Vitamin B2 (riboflavin) - 0.125 mg Pantothenic Acid - 0.393 mg Vitamin B6 - 0.278 mg Folate - 94 mcg Vitamin A - 1209 IU Vitamin E - 0.67

		Also contains small amounts of other minerals.	mg Vitamin K - 218.9 mcg Contains some other vitamins in small amounts.
Butternut squash 	One cup of Butternut squash, cooked, baked, drained with no added salt has 1.84 grams protein and 82 calories.	Potassium - 582 mg Phosphorus - 55 mg Magnesium - 59 mg Calcium - 84 mg Iron - 1.23 mg Zinc - 0.27 mg Copper - 0.133 mg Manganese - 0.353 mg Selenium - 1 mcg Sodium - 8 mg Also contains small amounts of other minerals.	Vitamin C - 31 mg Niacin - 1.986 mg Vitamin B1 (thiamine) - 0.148 mg Vitamin B2 (riboflavin) - 0.035 mg Pantothenic Acid - 0.736 mg Vitamin B6 - 0.254 mg Folate - 39 mcg Vitamin A - 22868 IU Vitamin K - 2 mcg Vitamin E - 2.64 mg Contains some other vitamins in small amounts.
Cabbage 	One half cup of cabbage, cooked, boiled, drained with no added salt has 0.95 grams protein, 17 calories and 1.4 grams of dietary fiber.	Potassium - 147 mg Phosphorus - 25 mg Magnesium - 11 mg Calcium - 36 mg Iron - 0.13 mg Sodium - 6 mg Zinc - 0.15 mg Copper - 0.013 mg Manganese - 0.154 mg Selenium - 0.5 mcg Also contains small amounts of other minerals.	Vitamin C - 28.1 mg Niacin - 0.186 mg Vitamin B1 (thiamine) - 0.046 mg Vitamin B2 (riboflavin) - 0.029 mg Vitamin B6 - 0.084 mg Folate - 22 mcg Pantothenic Acid - 0.13 mg Vitamin A - 60 IU Vitamin K - 81.5 mcg Vitamin E - 0.11 mg Contains some other vitamins in small amounts.
Carrots 	Half cup cooked with no added salt contains 0.59 grams protein, 27 calories and	Potassium - 183 mg Calcium - 23 mg Phosphorus - 23 mg Magnesium - 8 mg	Vitamin A - 13286 IU Vitamin C - 2.8 mg Vitamin B1 (thiamine) - 0.051 mg Vitamin

	2.3 grams fiber.	Iron - 0.27 mg Sodium - 5 mg Zinc - 0.3 mg Copper - 0.052 mg Manganese - 0.062 mg Selenium - 0.2 mcg Also contains small amounts of other minerals.	B2 (riboflavin) - 0.034 mg Niacin - 0.503 mg Folate - 11 mcg Pantothenic Acid - 0.181 mg Vitamin B6 - 0.119 mg Vitamin K - 10.7 mcg Vitamin E - 0.8 mg Contains some other vitamins in small amounts.
Cauliflower	Half cup cooked with no added salt contains 1.14 grams protein, 14 calories and 1.4 grams fiber.	Potassium - 88 mg Phosphorus - 20 mg Calcium - 10 mg Iron - 0.2 mg Magnesium - 6 mg Sodium - 9 mg Zinc - 0.11 mg Copper - 0.011 mg Manganese - 0.082 mg Selenium - 0.4 mcg Also contains small amounts of other minerals.	Vitamin C - 27.5 mg Niacin - 0.254 mg Vitamin B1 (thiamine) - 0.026 mg Vitamin B2 (riboflavin) - 0.032 mg Folate - 27 mcg Vitamin B6 - 0.107 mg Pantothenic Acid - 0.315 mg Vitamin A - 7 IU Vitamin K - 8.6 mcg Vitamin E - 0.04 mg Contains some other vitamins in small amounts.
Celeriac	One cup of Celeriac, cooked, boiled, drained with no added salt has 1.49 grams protein, 42 calories and 1.9 grams of dietary fiber.	Potassium - 268 mg Phosphorus - 102 mg Magnesium - 19 mg Calcium - 40 mg Iron - 0.67 mg Sodium - 95 mg Zinc - 0.31 mg Copper - 0.067 mg Manganese - 0.149 mg Selenium - 0.6 mcg Also contains small amounts of other minerals.	Vitamin C - 5.6 mg Niacin - 0.662 mg Vitamin B1 (thiamine) - 0.042 mg Vitamin B2 (riboflavin) - 0.057 mg Vitamin B6 - 0.157 mg Folate - 5 mcg Pantothenic Acid - 0.315 mg Contains some other vitamins in small amounts.
Celery	One cup of celery,	Potassium - 426 mg	Vitamin C - 9.2 mg Niacin - 0.479 mg

	cooked, boiled, drained with no added salt has 1.25 grams protein, 27 calories and 2.4 grams of dietary fiber.	Phosphorus - 38 mg Magnesium - 18 mg Calcium - 63 mg Iron - 0.63 mg Sodium - 136 mg Zinc - 0.21 mg Copper - 0.054 mg Manganese - 0.159 mg Selenium - 1.5 mcg Also contains small amounts of other minerals.	Vitamin B1 (thiamine) - 0.064 mg Vitamin B2 (riboflavin) - 0.07 mg Vitamin B6 - 0.129 mg Folate - 33 mcg Pantothenic Acid - 0.292 mg Vitamin A - 782 IU Vitamin K - 56.7 mcg Vitamin E - 0.53 IU Contains some other vitamins in small amounts.
Chinese broccoli 	One cup of Chinese broccoli, cooked, boiled, drained with no added salt has 1 gram protein, 19 calories and 2.2 grams of dietary fiber.	Potassium - 230 mg Phosphorus - 36 mg Magnesium - 16 mg Calcium - 88 mg Iron - 0.49 mg Sodium - 6 mg Zinc - 0.34 mg Copper - 0.054 mg Manganese - 0.232 mg Selenium - 1.1 mcg Also contains small amounts of other minerals.	Vitamin C - 24.8 mg Niacin - 0.385 mg Vitamin B1 (thiamine) - 0.084 mg Vitamin B2 (riboflavin) - 0.128 mg Vitamin B6 - 0.062 mg Folate - 87 mcg Pantothenic Acid - 0.14 mg Vitamin A - 1441 IU Vitamin K - 74.6 mcg Vitamin E - 0.42 mg Contains some other vitamins in small amounts.
Chinese cabbage 	One cup of Chinese cabbage (pe-tsai), cooked, boiled, drained with no added salt has 1.78 grams protein, 17 calories and 2 grams of dietary fiber.	Potassium - 268 mg Phosphorus - 46 mg Magnesium - 12 mg Calcium - 38 mg Iron - 0.36 mg Sodium - 11 mg Zinc - 0.21 mg Copper - 0.035 mg Manganese - 0.182 mg Selenium - 0.5 mcg Also contains	Vitamin C - 18.8 mg Niacin - 0.595 mg Vitamin B1 (thiamine) - 0.052 mg Vitamin B2 (riboflavin) - 0.052 mg Vitamin B6 - 0.0211 mg Folate - 63 mcg Pantothenic Acid - 0.095 mg Vitamin A - 1151 IU Contains some other vitamins in

		small amounts of other minerals.	small amounts.
Corn	One large ear of yellow corn, cooked with no salt contains 4.02 grams protein, 113 calories and 2.8 grams fiber.	Potassium - 257 mg Phosphorus - 91 mg Magnesium - 31 mg Calcium - 4 mg Selenium - 0.2 mg Iron - 0.53 mg Zinc - 0.73 mg Copper - 0.058 mg Manganese - 0.197 mg Also contains small amounts of other minerals.	Vitamin C - 6.5 mg Niacin - 1.986 mg Vitamin B1 (thiamine) - 0.11 mg Vitamin B2 (riboflavin) - 0.067 mg Vitamin B6 - 0.164 mg Folate - 27 mcg Pantothenic Acid - 0.935 mg Vitamin A - 310 IU Vitamin K - 0.5 mcg Vitamin E - 0.11 mg Contains some other vitamins in small amounts.
Cucumber	Half a cup of sliced cucumber with skins contains .34 grams protein, 8 calories and .3 grams fiber.	Potassium - 76 mg Phosphorus - 12 mg Magnesium - 7 mg Sodium - 1 mg Calcium - 8 mg Iron - 0.15 mg Zinc - 0.1 mg Copper - 0.021 mg Manganese - 0.041 mg Selenium - 0.2 mcg Also contains small amounts of other minerals.	Vitamin C - 1.5 mg Niacin - 0.051 mg Vitamin B1 (thiamine) - 0.014 mg Vitamin B2 (riboflavin) - 0.017 mg Vitamin B6 - 0.021 mg Folate - 4 mcg Pantothenic Acid - 0.135 mg Vitamin A - 55 IU Vitamin K - 8.5 mcg Vitamin E - 0.02 mg Contains some other vitamins in small amounts.
Daikon Radish	One cup of Daikon Radish(oriental), cooked, boiled, drained with no added salt has 0.98 grams protein, 25 calories and 2.4 grams of dietary fiber.	Potassium - 419 mg Phosphorus - 35 mg Magnesium - 13 mg Calcium - 25 mg Iron - 0.22 mg < Sodium - 19 mg Zinc - 0.19 mg Copper - 0.148 mg Manganese - 0.049 mg	Vitamin C - 22.2 mg Niacin - 0.221 mg Vitamin B2 (riboflavin) - 0.034 mg Vitamin B6 - 0.056 mg Folate - 25 mcg Pantothenic Acid - 0.168 mg Vitamin K - 0.4 mcg Contains some other vitamins in

		Selenium - 1 mcg Also contains small amounts of other minerals.	small amounts.
Eggplant	One cup of eggplant, cooked, boiled, drained with no added salt has 0.82 grams protein, 35 calories and 2.5 grams of dietary fiber.	Potassium - 122 mg Phosphorus - 15 mg Magnesium - 11 mg Calcium - 6 mg Iron - 0.25 mg Sodium - 1 mg Zinc - 0.12 mg Copper - 0.058 mg Manganese - 0.112 mg Selenium - 0.1 mcg Also contains small amounts of other minerals.	Vitamin C - 1.3 mg Niacin - 0.594 mg Vitamin B1 (thiamine) - 0.075 mg Vitamin B2 (riboflavin) - 0.02 mg Vitamin B6 - 0.085 mg Folate - 14 mcg Pantothenic Acid - 0.074 mg Vitamin A - 37 IU Vitamin K - 2.9 mcg Vitamin E - 0.41 mg Contains some other vitamins in small amounts.
Fennel	One cup of raw fennel bulb has 1.08 grams protein, 27 calories and 2.7 grams of dietary fiber.	Potassium - 360 mg Phosphorus - 44 mg Magnesium - 15 mg Calcium - 43 mg Iron - 0.64 mg Sodium - 45 mg Zinc - 0.17 mg Copper - 0.057 mg Manganese - 0.166 mg Selenium - 0.6 mcg Also contains small amounts of other minerals.	Vitamin C - 10.4 mg Niacin - 0.557 mg Vitamin B1 (thiamine) - 0.009 mg Vitamin B2 (riboflavin) - 0.028 mg Vitamin B6 - 0.041 mg Folate - 23 mcg Pantothenic Acid - 0.202 mg Vitamin A - 117 IU Contains some other vitamins in small amounts.
French beans	One cup of French beans, mature seeds, cooked, boiled with no added salt has 12.48 grams protein, 228 calories and	Potassium - 655 mg Phosphorus - 181 mg Magnesium - 99 mg Calcium - 112 mg Iron - 1.91 mg Sodium - 11 mg Zinc - 1.13 mg Copper - 0.204	Vitamin C - 2.1 mg Niacin - 0.966 mg Vitamin B1 (thiamine) - 0.23 mg Vitamin B2 (riboflavin) - 0.11 mg Vitamin B6 - 0.186 mg Folate - 133 mcg Pantothenic Acid -

	16.6 grams of dietary fiber.	mg Manganese - 0.676 mg Selenium - 2.1 mcg Also contains small amounts of other minerals.	0.393 mg Vitamin A - 5 IU Contains some other vitamins in small amounts.
Jicama	One hundred grams of jicama, cooked or boiled with no added salt has 0.72 grams protein and 38 calories.	Potassium - 135 mg Phosphorus - 16 mg Magnesium - 11 mg Calcium - 11 mg Iron - 0.57 mg Sodium - 4 mg Zinc - 0.15 mg Copper - 0.046 mg Manganese - 0.057 mg Selenium - 0.7 mcg Also contains small amounts of other minerals.	Vitamin C - 14.1 mg Niacin - 0.19 mg Vitamin B1 (thiamine) - 0.017 mg Vitamin B2 (riboflavin) - 0.028 mg Vitamin B6 - 0.04 mg Folate - 8 mcg Pantothenic Acid - 0.121 mg Vitamin A - 19 IU Contains some other vitamins in small amounts.
Kale	One cup of cooked kale with no added salt contains 2.47 grams protein, 36 calories and 2.6 grams fiber.	Potassium - 296 mg Phosphorus - 36 mg Magnesium - 23 mg Calcium - 94 mg Iron - 1.17 mg Sodium - 30 mg Zinc - 0.31 mg Copper - 0.203 mg Manganese - 0.541 mg Selenium - 1.2 mcg Also contains small amounts of other minerals.	Vitamin A - 17,707 IU Vitamin C - 53.3 mg Niacin - 0.65 mg Vitamin B1 (thiamine) - 0.069 mg Vitamin B2 (riboflavin) - 0.091 mg Vitamin B6 - 0.179 mg Folate - 17 mcg Pantothenic Acid - 0.064 mg Vitamin K - 1062 mcg Vitamin E - 1.1 mg Contains some other vitamins in small amounts.
Leek	One leek, cooked, boiled with no added salt has 1 gram protein, 38 calories and	Potassium - 108 mg Phosphorus - 21 mg Magnesium - 17 mg Calcium - 37 mg	Vitamin C - 5.2 mg Niacin - 0.248 mg Vitamin B1 (thiamine) - 0.032 mg Vitamin B2 (riboflavin) -

	1.2 grams of dietary fiber.	Iron - 1.36 mg Sodium - 12 mg Zinc - 0.07 mg Copper - 0.077 mg Manganese - 0.306 mg Selenium - 0.6 mcg Also contains small amounts of other minerals.	0.025 mg Vitamin B6 - 0.14 mg Folate - 30 mcg Pantothenic Acid - 0.089 mg Vitamin A - 1007 IU Vitamin K - 31.5 mcg Vitamin E - 0.62 mg Contains some other vitamins in small amounts.
Lima Beans	One cup of cooked large lima beans with no added salt contains 14.66 grams protein, 216 calories and 13.2 grams fiber.	Potassium - 955 mg Phosphorus - 209 mg Magnesium - 81 mg Calcium - 32 mg Selenium - 8.5 mg Iron - 4.49 mg Sodium - 4 mg Zinc - 1.79 mg Manganese - 0.97 mg Copper - 0.442 mg Also contains small amounts of other minerals.	Pantothenic Acid - 0.793 mg Niacin - 0.791 mg Vitamin B1 (thiamine) - 0.303 mg Vitamin B2 (riboflavin) - 0.103 mg Vitamin B6 - 0.303 mg Folate - 156 mcg Vitamin K - 3.8 mcg Vitamin E - 0.34 mg Contains some other vitamins in small amounts.
Mushroom	Half a cup of raw mushrooms contains 1.08 grams of protein, 8 calories and 0.3 grams of fiber.	Potassium - 111 mg Phosphorus - 30 mg Magnesium - 3 mg Calcium - 1 mg Iron - 0.17 mg Sodium - 2 mg Zinc - 0.18 mg Copper - 0.111 mg Manganese - 0.016 mg Selenium - 3.3 mcg Also contains small amounts of other minerals.	Vitamin D - 2 IU Niacin - 1.262 mg Vitamin B1 (thiamine) - 0.028 mg Vitamin B2 (riboflavin) - 0.141 mg Vitamin B6 - 0.036 mg Vitamin C - 0.7 mg Pantothenic Acid - 0.524 mg Folate - 6 mcg Contains some other vitamins in small amounts.
Okra	One cup of okra, cooked, boiled, drained, with	Potassium - 216 mg Phosphorus - 51 mg	Vitamin C - 26.1 mg Niacin - 1.394 mg Vitamin

	no added salt has 3 grams protein, 35 calories and 4 grams of dietary fiber.	Magnesium - 58 mg Calcium - 123 mg Iron - 0.45 mg Sodium - 10 mg Zinc - 0.69 mg Copper - 0.136 mg Manganese - 0.47 mg Selenium - 0.6 mcg Also contains small amounts of other minerals.	B1 (thiamine) - 0.211 mg Vitamin B2 (riboflavin) - 0.088 mg Vitamin B6 - 0.299 mg Folate - 74 mcg Pantothenic Acid - 0.341 mg Vitamin A - 453 IU Vitamin K - 64 mcg Vitamin E - 0.43 mg Contains some other vitamins in small amounts.
Onions 	One small onion cooked without salt contains 0.82 grams protein, 26 calories and 0.8 grams of fiber.	Potassium - 100 mg Phosphorus - 21 mg Calcium - 13 mg Iron - 0.14 mg Magnesium - 7 mg Sodium - 2 mg Zinc - 0.13 mg Copper - 0.04 mg Manganese - 0.092 mg Selenium - 0.4 mcg Also contains small amounts other minerals.	Vitamin C - 3.1 mg Niacin - 0.099 mg Vitamin B1 (thiamine) - 0.025 mg Vitamin B2 (riboflavin) - 0.014 mg Vitamin B6 - 0.077 mg Pantothenic Acid - 0.068 mg Folate - 9 mcg Vitamin A - 1 IU Vitamin K - 0.3 mcg Vitamin E - 0.01 mg Contains some other vitamins in small amounts.
Parsnip 	One cup of parsnip, cooked, boiled, drained, with no added salt has 2.06 grams protein, 111 calories and 5.6 grams of dietary fiber.	Potassium - 573 mg Phosphorus - 108 mg Magnesium - 45 mg Calcium - 58 mg Iron - 0.9 mg Sodium - 16 mg Zinc - 0.41 mg Copper - 0.215 mg Manganese - 0.459 mg Selenium - 2.7 mcg Also contains small amounts of other minerals.	Vitamin C - 20.3 mg Niacin - 1.129 mg Vitamin B1 (thiamine) - 0.129 mg Vitamin B2 (riboflavin) - 0.08 mg Vitamin B6 - 0.145 mg Folate - 90 mcg Pantothenic Acid - 0.917 mg Vitamin K - 1.6 mcg Vitamin E - 1.56 mg Contains some other vitamins in small amounts.

Peas	One cup of boiled peas with no salt added contains 8.58 grams of protein, 134 calories and 8.8 grams of fiber.	Potassium - 434 mg Phosphorus - 187 mg Magnesium - 62 mg Calcium - 43 mg Sodium - 5 mg Selenium - 3.0 mg Iron - 2.46 mg Zinc - 1.9 mg Manganese - 0.84 mg Copper - 0.277 mg Also contains small amounts of other minerals.	Vitamin A - 1282 IU Vitamin C - 22.7 mg Niacin - 3.234 mg Folate - 101 mcg Vitamin B1 (thiamine) - 0.414 mg Vitamin B2 (riboflavin) - 0.238 mg Vitamin B6 - 0.346 mg Pantothenic Acid - 0.245 mg Vitamin K - 41.4 mcg Vitamin E - 0.22 mg Contains some other vitamins in small amounts.
Potatoes	One medium baked potato without salt contains 4.33 grams of protein, 161 calories and 3.8 grams of fiber.	Potassium - 926 mg Phosphorus - 121 mg Magnesium - 48 mg Calcium - 26 mg Iron - 1.87 mg Sodium - 17 mg Zinc - 0.62 mg Copper - 0.204 mg Manganese - 0.379 mg Selenium - 0.7 mcg Also contains small amounts of other minerals.	Vitamin C - 16.6 mg Niacin - 2.439 mg Vitamin B1 (thiamine) - 0.111 mg Vitamin B2 (riboflavin) - 0.083 mg Pantothenic Acid - 0.65 mg Vitamin B6 - 0.538 mg Folate - 48 mcg Vitamin A - 17 IU Vitamin K - 3.5 mcg Vitamin E - 0.07 mg Contains some other vitamins in small amounts.
Pumpkin	One cup of pumpkin, cooked, boiled, drained, with no added salt has 1.76 grams protein, 49 calories and 2.7 grams of dietary fiber.	Potassium - 564 mg Phosphorus - 74 mg Magnesium - 22 mg Calcium - 37 mg Iron - 1.4 mg Sodium - 2 mg Zinc - 0.56 mg Copper - 0.223 mg Manganese - 0.218 mg	Vitamin C - 11.5 mg Niacin - 1.012 mg Vitamin B1 (thiamine) - 0.076 mg Vitamin B2 (riboflavin) - 0.191 mg Vitamin B6 - 0.108 mg Folate - 22 mcg Pantothenic Acid - 0.492 mg

		Selenium - 0.5 mcg Also contains small amounts of other minerals.	Vitamin A - 12230 IU Vitamin K - 2 mcg Vitamin E - 1.96 mg Contains some other vitamins in small amounts.
Radish	One half cup of radishes, raw, has 0.39 grams protein, 9 calories and 0.9 grams of dietary fiber.	Potassium - 135 mg Phosphorus - 12 mg Magnesium - 6 mg Calcium - 14 mg Iron - 0.2 mg Sodium - 23 mg Zinc - 0.16 mg Copper - 0.029 mg Manganese - 0.04 mg Selenium - 0.3 mcg Also contains small amounts of other minerals.	Vitamin C - 8.6 mg Niacin - 0.147 mg Vitamin B1 (thiamine) - 0.007 mg Vitamin B2 (riboflavin) - 0.023 mg Vitamin B6 - 0.041 mg Folate - 14 mcg Pantothenic Acid - 0.096 mg Vitamin A - 4 IU Vitamin K - 0.8 mcg Contains some other vitamins in small amounts.
Rapini	One cup of rapini, raw, has 1.27 grams protein, 9 calories and 1.1 grams of dietary fiber.	Potassium - 78 mg Phosphorus - 29 mg Magnesium - 9 mg Calcium - 43 mg Iron - 0.86 mg Sodium - 13 mg Zinc - 0.31 mg Copper - 0.017 mg Manganese - 0.158 mg Selenium - 0.4 mcg Also contains small amounts of other minerals.	Vitamin C - 8.1 mg Niacin - 0.488 mg Vitamin B1 (thiamine) - 0.065 mg Vitamin B2 (riboflavin) - 0.052 mg Vitamin B6 - 0.068 mg Folate - 33 mcg Pantothenic Acid - 0.129 mg Vitamin A - 1049 IU Vitamin K - 89.6 mcg Vitamin E - 0.65 mg Contains some other vitamins in small amounts.
Spinach	One cup of raw spinach contains 0.86 grams of protein, 7 calories and 0.7 grams of fiber.	Potassium - 167 mg Phosphorus - 15 mg Magnesium - 24 mg Calcium - 30 mg Iron - 0.81 mg	Vitamin C - 8.4 mg Niacin - 0.217 mg Vitamin B1 (thiamine) - 0.023 mg Vitamin B2 (riboflavin) - 0.057 mg

		Sodium - 24 mg Zinc - 0.16 mg Copper - 0.039 mg Manganese - 0.269 mg Selenium - 0.3 mcg Also contains small amounts of other minerals.	Vitamin B6 - 0.059 mg Pantothenic Acid - 0.02 mg Folate - 58 mcg Vitamin A - 2813 mg Vitamin K - 144.9 mcg Vitamin E - 0.61 mg Contains some other vitamins in small amounts.
Spirulina (seaweed)	One cup of dried spirulina has 64.37 grams protein, 325 calories and 4 grams of dietary fiber.	Potassium - 1527 mg Phosphorus - 132 mg Magnesium - 218 mg Calcium - 134 mg Iron - 31.92 mg Zinc - 2.24 mg Manganese - 2.128 mg Sodium - 1174 mg Selenium - 8.1 mg Copper - 6.832 mg Also contains small amounts of other minerals.	Vitamin C - 11.3 mg Niacin - 14.358 mg Vitamin B1 (thiamine) - 2.666 mg Vitamin B2 (riboflavin) - 4.11 mg Vitamin B6 - 0.408 mg Pantothenic Acid - 3.898 mg Folate - 105 mcg Vitamin A - 638 mg Vitamin K - 28.6 mcg Vitamin E - 5.6 mg Contains some other vitamins in small amounts.
Spaghetti squash	One cup of spaghetti squash, cooked, boiled, drained, and with no added salt contains 1.02 grams protein, 42 calories and 2.2 grams of dietary fiber.	Potassium - 181 mg Phosphorus - 22 mg Magnesium - 17 mg Calcium - 33 mg Iron - 0.53 mg Sodium - 28 mg Zinc - 0.31 mg Copper - 0.054 mg Manganese - 0.169 mg Selenium - 0.5 mcg Also contains small amounts of other minerals.	Vitamin C - 5.4 mg Niacin - 1.256 mg Vitamin B1 (thiamine) - 0.059 mg Vitamin B2 (riboflavin) - 0.034 mg Vitamin B6 - 0.153 mg Pantothenic Acid - 0.55 mg Folate - 12 mcg Vitamin A - 170 mg Vitamin K - 1.2 mcg Vitamin E - 0.19 mg Contains some other vitamins in small amounts.
Squash, Summer	One cup of	Potassium - 319	Vitamin C - 20.9

	sliced summer squash, boiled with no added salt contains 1.87 grams of protein, 41 calories and 2 grams of fiber.	mg Phosphorus - 52 mg Magnesium - 29 mg Calcium - 40 mg Sodium - 2 mg Iron - 0.67 mg Manganese - 0.283 mg Selenium - 0.4 mg Zinc - 0.4 mg Copper - 0.117 mg Also contains small amounts of other minerals.	mg Niacin - .913 mg Vitamin B1 (thiamine) - 0.077 mg Vitamin B2 (riboflavin) - 0.045 mg Vitamin B6 - 0.14 mg Pantothenic Acid - 0.581 mg Folate - 41 mcg Vitamin A - 2011 mg Vitamin K - 7.9 mcg Vitamin E - 0.22 mg Contains some other vitamins in small amounts.
Squash, Winter	One cup of cubed winter squash, baked with no added salt contains 1.82 grams of protein, 76 calories and 5.7 grams of fiber.	Potassium - 494 mg Phosphorus - 39 mg Magnesium - 27 mg Calcium - 45 mg Sodium - 2 mg Iron - 0.9 mg Zinc - 0.45 mg Copper - 0.168 mg Manganese - 0.383 mg Selenium - 0.8 mcg Also contains small amounts of other minerals.	Vitamin C - 19.7 mg Niacin - 1.015 mg Vitamin B1 (thiamine) - 0.033 mg Vitamin B2 (riboflavin) - 0.137 mg Vitamin B6 - 0.33 mg Folate - 41 mcg Pantothenic Acid - 0.48 mg Vitamin A - 10707 mg Vitamin K - 9 mcg Vitamin E - 0.25 mg Contains some other vitamins in small amounts.
Sweet Potatoes	One medium sweet potato baked in its skin contains 2.29 grams of protein, 103 calories and 3.8 grams of fiber.	Potassium - 542 mg Phosphorus - 62 mg Magnesium - 31 mg Calcium - 43 mg Sodium - 41 mg Iron - 0.79 mg Selenium - 0.2 mg Manganese - 0.567 mg Zinc - 0.36 mg	Vitamin C - 22.3 mg Niacin - 1.695 mg Vitamin B1 (thiamine) - 0.122 mg Vitamin B2 (riboflavin) - 0.121 mg Vitamin B6 - 0.326 mg Pantothenic Acid - 1.008 mg Folate - 7 mcg

		Copper - 0.184 mg Also contains small amounts of other minerals.	Vitamin A - 21,909 mg Vitamin K - 2.6 mcg Vitamin E - 0.81 mg Contains some other vitamins in small amounts.
Swiss chard	One cup of Swiss chard, cooked, boiled, drained, has 3.29 grams protein, 35 calories and 3.7 grams of dietary fiber.	Potassium - 961 mg Phosphorus - 58 mg Magnesium - 150 mg Calcium - 102 mg Iron - 3.95 mg Sodium - 313 mg Zinc - 0.58 mg Copper - 0.285 mg Manganese - 0.585 mg Selenium - 1.6 mcg Also contains small amounts of other minerals.	Vitamin C - 31.5 mg Niacin - 0.63 mg Vitamin B1 (thiamine) - 0.06 mg Vitamin B2 (riboflavin) - 0.15 mg Vitamin B6 - 0.149 mg Pantothenic Acid - 0.285 mg Folate - 16 mcg Vitamin A - 10717 IU Vitamin K - 572.8 mcg Vitamin E - 3.31 mg Contains some other vitamins in small amounts.
Taro	One cup of taro, raw, has 1.56 grams protein, 116 calories and 4.3 grams of dietary fiber.	Potassium - 615 mg Phosphorus - 87 mg Magnesium - 34 mg Calcium - 45 mg Iron - 0.57 mg Sodium - 11 mg Zinc - 0.24 mg Copper - 0.179 mg Manganese - 0.398 mg Selenium - 0.7 mcg Also contains small amounts of other minerals.	Vitamin C - 4.7 mg Niacin - 0.624 mg Vitamin B1 (thiamine) - 0.099 mg Vitamin B2 (riboflavin) - 0.026 mg Vitamin B6 - 0.294 mg Folate - 23 mcg Pantothenic Acid - 0.315 mg Vitamin A - 79 IU Vitamin K - 1 mcg Vitamin E - 2.48 mg Contains some other vitamins in small amounts.
Turnip	One cup of turnips, boiled with no added salt, has 1.11	Potassium - 276 mg Phosphorus - 41 mg Magnesium - 14	Vitamin C - 18.1 mg Niacin - 0.466 mg Vitamin B1 (thiamine) -

	grams protein, 34 calories and 3.1 grams of dietary fiber.	mg Calcium - 51 mg Iron - 0.28 mg Zinc - 0.19 mg Copper - 0.003 mg Manganese - 0.111 mg Selenium - 0.3 mcg Also contains small amounts other minerals.	0.042 mg Vitamin B2 (riboflavin) - 0.036 mg Vitamin B6 - 0.105 mg Pantothenic Acid - 0.222 mg Folate - 14 mcg Vitamin K - 0.2 mcg Vitamin E - 0.03 mg Contains some other vitamins in small amounts.
Yellow squash	One cup of yellow (crookneck) squash, raw, has 1.28 grams protein, 24 calories and 1.3 grams of dietary fiber.	Potassium - 282 mg Phosphorus - 41 mg Magnesium - 25 mg Calcium - 27 mg Iron - 0.56 mg Sodium - 3 mg Zinc - 0.37 mg Copper - 0.117 mg Manganese - 0.218 mg Selenium - 0.3 mcg Also contains small amounts of other minerals.	Vitamin C - 24.5 mg Niacin - 0.569 mg Vitamin B1 (thiamine) - 0.065 mg Vitamin B2 (riboflavin) - 0.052 mg Vitamin B6 - 0.132 mg Folate - 24 mcg Pantothenic Acid - 0.203 mg Vitamin A - 190 IU Vitamin K - 4.1 mcg Vitamin E - 0.17 mg Contains some other vitamins in small amounts.

You can see from the table above that there really are a large variety of delicious and healthy vegetables available for you to eat and enjoy throughout the year! All these vegetables will provide your body with a continuous alkalizing and healing effect in different degrees and they can be cooked with a myriad of tasty recipes that suit your preferences.

Chapter 3

Cancer's Favorite Food

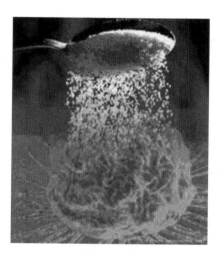

In the first chapter you've learned about an amazing discovery by Dr. Otto Warburg. Way back in 1924 Dr. Otto Warburg discovered the main biochemical cause of cancer, or what **differentiates a cancer cell** from a normal, **healthy cell**. Dr. Otto Warburg was actually awarded the Nobel Prize for this big discovery.

Cancer has only one prime cause. It is the replacement of normal oxygen respiration of the body's cells by an anaerobic [i.e., oxygen-deficient] cell respiration. -Dr. Otto Warburg

What else does Warburg's discovery tell us? It tells us that cancer **metabolizes** much differently than normal cells. Normal cells need oxygen. Cancer cells despise oxygen.

Another thing this tells us is that cancer metabolizes through a process of fermentation.

Warburg was the first to describe in detail the **dependence** of **cancer cells** on **glucose** and **glycolysis** in order to maintain viability following irreversible respiratory damage. He considered **respiration** and **fermentation** as the sole producers of **energy within cells**, and energy alone as the central issue of tumorigenesis.

"We need to know no more of respiration and fermentation here than that they are energy-producing reactions and that they synthesize the energy-rich adenosine triphosphate, through which the energy of respiration and fermentation is then made available for life" Dr. Otto Warburg.

If you've ever made wine, you'll know that fermentation requires **sugar**.

The metabolism of cancer is approximately 8 times greater than the metabolism of normal cells.

The body is constantly overworked **trying to feed cancer**. The cancer is constantly on the verge of starvation and thus constantly asking the body to feed it. When the food supply is cut off, the cancer begins to starve unless it can make the body produce sugar to feed itself.

The wasting syndrome, **cachexia** is the body producing sugar from proteins (you heard it right, not from carbohydrates or fats, but from proteins) in a process called glycogenesis. **This sugar feeds the cancer**. The body finally dies of starvation, **trying to feed the cancer**.

Now, knowing that one's cancer needs sugar, does it make sense to feed it sugar? Does it make sense to have a high carbohydrate diet?

The reason Food Therapies for cancer even exist today (beyond the fact that they work) is because someone once saw the **connection between sugar and cancer**. There are many food therapies, but not a single one allows many foods high in carbohydrates and not a single one allows sugars, **BECAUSE SUGAR FEEDS CANCER.**

Sugary drinks kill 180,000 people annually through diabetes, cancer and heart disease, a recent Harvard study claims

Sugary drinks aren't just fattening - they're deadly, according to a new study out of **Harvard**.
The study links roughly 180,000 deaths annually in the USA to sugar-sweetened beverages, including **soda, sports drinks** and **fruit drinks**.
Specifically, sugary drinks are linked with 133,000 deaths from diabetes, **6,000 deaths from cancer**, and 44,000 deaths from heart disease worldwide.

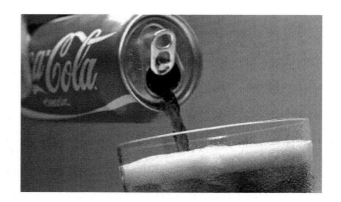

In the U.S. alone, the research shows that about 25,000 deaths in 2010 were linked to drinking sugar-sweetened beverages, said Gitanjali M. Singh, Ph.D., co-author of the study and a postdoctoral research fellow at the Harvard School of Public Health.

The study was presented on the 19 March 2013 at a meeting of the American Heart Association.

The health effects of drinking sugary beverages have been the topic of heated public debate across the country recently and especially in New York, where Mayor Michael Bloomberg has tried unsuccessfully to ban businesses from selling them in sizes larger than 16 ounces.

Bloomberg cited a number of studies linking sugary drink consumption to higher rates of obesity in making his argument for the ban, and he will likely add the new Harvard study to the pile as he fights for an appeal.

The Harvard researchers scrubbed data from a 2010 Global Burden of Diseases study on the consumption levels of sugar-sweetened drinks to measure global intake.
The results revealed that geography may have an impact on how sugary drinks affect certain populations.

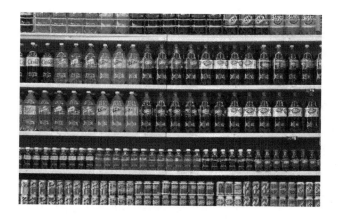

Of nine world regions, Latin American and Caribbean countries had the most diabetes-related deaths associated with sugary drinks, while East and Central Europe/Asia claimed the most heart-related deaths.

Overall, among the world's 15 most populous countries, Mexico had the highest rate of deaths associated with sugary drink consumption, with roughly 317 deaths for every million adults.

You might be thinking that you are consuming drinks that have **"0 Sugar"** or **"NO sugar"**. And why do you think there is not much difference in taste and they still sweet? The answer is **Artificial Sweeteners** and one of them is a very dangerous one by the name of **Aspartame**.

Study: Aspartame linked to blood cancers

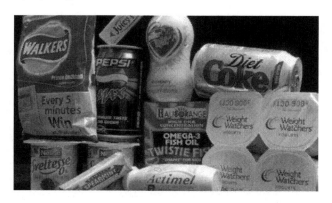

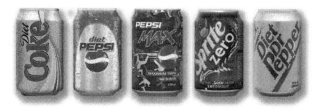

A new human study shows that aspartame use is linked to increased risk of leukemia, non-Hodgkin lymphoma (NHL), and multiple myeloma in men.

A newly published long term study that spans 22 years shows that drinking one or more **aspartame-sweetened** soft drinks per day increases the risk of several blood cancers in men. The study was led by Dr. Eva S. Schernhammer of the Channing Division of Network Medicine, Department of Medicine, Brigham and Women's Hospital and Harvard Medical School in Boston.

Men who consumed one or more aspartame-sweetened sodas per day had an increased risk of NHL and multiple myeloma, compared to men who didn't drink diet soda. This study was published in *The American Journal of Clinical Nutrition.*

The Prime Cause and Prevention of Cancer   with two prefaces on prevention

Revised lecture at the meeting of the Nobel Laureates on June 30, 1966 at Lindau, Lake Constance, Germany

By Dr.   Otto Warburg   Director, Max Planck-Institute for Cell Physiology, Berlin-Dahlem

English Edition by Dean Burk   National Cancer Institute, Bethesda, Maryland, USA

"... **for cancer, there is only one prime cause. Summarized in a few words, the prime cause of cancer is the replacement of the respiration of oxygen in normal body cells by FERMENTATION OF SUGAR. All normal body cells meet their energy needs by RESPIRATION OF OXYGEN, whereas cancer cells meet their energy needs in great part by FERMENTATION.**

In every case, during the cancer development, the oxygen respiration always falls, FERMENTATION appears, and the highly differentiated cells are transformed into fermenting anaerobes, which have lost all their body functions and retain only the now useless

property of growth and replication. Thus, when respiration disappears, life does not disappear, but the meaning of life disappears, and what remains are growing machines that destroy the body in which they grow..."

The average American consumes an astounding 2-3 pounds of sugar each week, which is not surprising considering that highly refined sugars in the form of **sucrose** (table sugar), **dextrose** (corn sugar), **high-fructose corn syrup** (HFCS), **corn syrup** etc. are being processed into so many foods such as bread, cereals, ketchup, mayonnaise, peanut butter, salad dressings, jams, sauces, premade meals etc.

In the last 20 years **sugar consumption** only in US was increased from **26 pounds** to **135 pounds** per person per Year!
The average consumption 1887-1890 was only **5 pounds** per person per year!

According to the American Cancer Society, **Forty-one thousand (41,000)** Americans (64 people per 100,000) died of cancer in 1900.

Nowadays each year globally, **12.7 million** people learn they have cancer, and **7.6 million** people die from cancer.

Cancer is the **second** leading cause of **death** in the United States, exceeded only by heart disease.

It kills over **1,500 U.S. citizens every day**. And it kills nearly 547,500 Americans in a single year; that number is rising.

Researchers at Huntsman Cancer Institute in Utah were one of the first to discover that **sugar "feeds" tumors**. The research published in the journal *Proceedings of the National Academy of Sciences* said, "It's been known since 1923 that tumor cells use a lot more glucose than normal cells. Our research helps show how this process takes place, and how it might be stopped to control tumor growth," says Don Ayer, Ph.D., a professor in the Department of Oncological Sciences at the University of Utah.

Dr. Thomas Graeber, a professor of molecular and medical pharmacology, has investigated how the metabolism of glucose affects the biochemical signals present in cancer cells. In research published June 26, 2012 in the journal *Molecular Systems Biology*, Graeber and his colleagues demonstrate that **glucose starvation—that is, depriving cancer cells of glucose—activates a metabolic and signaling amplification loop that <u>leads to cancer cell death</u>** as a result of the toxic accumulation of reactive oxygen species (ROS).

Drs. Rainer Klement and Ulrike Kammerer conducted a comprehensive review of the literature involving dietary carbohydrates and their **direct** and **indirect effect** on **cancer cells**, which was published in October 2011 in the journal ***Nutrition and Metabolism***, concluding that cancers are so sensitive to the sugar supply that cutting that supply will suppress cancer. **"Increased glucose flux and metabolism promotes several hallmarks of cancer such as excessive proliferation, anti-apoptotic signaling, cell cycle progression and angiogenesis."**

Eating white sugar, refined flower and processed food causes magnesium mineral deficiencies because the magnesium has been removed in the processing, **making sugar a ripe target as a major cause of cancer because deficiencies in magnesium are not only pro-inflammatory but also pro-cancer**.

I would like you to pay significant attention to the body's storing of fat.

The body stores body fat mainly for these 3 reasons:

1. Too many calories from **refined** and **processed carbohydrates** that strip away beneficial fiber or **bad fats.**

2. It is not getting the required **good healthy fats** it needs to run the body smoothly.

3. Interference in the action of the hormone **Leptin, which** plays a key role in our appetite.

The **first reason** is pretty simple. When we eat more than our body requires for energy it stores these excess calories as fat. This is the fat we see on our bellies, hips, and thighs. The fat most of us desperately want to get rid of.

The **second reason** our body stores fat is because it is not getting the required "good" fats it needs to run smoothly.

The **third reason** is when your brain doesn't get a signal that your stomach is full. I am sure many of you will recognize this feeling, like after eating a big meal you still feel hungry. And you think why? The reason is that leptin hormone which is responsible to give a signal to your brain that your tummy is full and there is no little space for food any more didn't do its crucial job and didn't deliver the signal. **Leptin is called the "satisfaction" hormone because it tells your brain that you've had enough to eat**. It can also tell the body to **burn more calories** based on how much you eat.

It is not your fault that you still feel hungry and wish to eat more even after a big meal.

One of the reasons for your brain not getting a message is when you consume food which includes **High Fructose Corn Syrup (HFCS).** You will be amazed to find out how much food contains HFCS when you start checking ingredients.

In a review of research, George Bray and colleagues at Louisiana State University found fructose doesn't trip the leptin sensor or promote enhanced production of leptin. In addition, after consuming **high-fructose corn syrup**, participants of some studies had reduced leptin concentrations. Other sweeteners, like glucose, provide satiety signals to the brain that fructose cannot provide, because it is **not transported into the brain**. In an animal study, a diet high in high-fructose corn syrup led to leptin resistance. This causes cells to stop accepting leptin's messages, regardless of how much leptin you have in your body. In both study sets, the results were **significant weight gain** and **habitual consumption of more calories**.

Research published in the December 2008 issue of the "American Journal of Clinical Nutrition" says that prolonged consumption of food and beverages containing fructose-based sweeteners can lead to both overeating and reduce calorie burning by your body. As a result, you can gain weight. Leptin works in the hypothalamus region of the brain, and research has demonstrated that your body's metabolism of high-fructose corn syrup may skip all of the processes that would trigger the work of leptin.

"A diet high in high fructose corn syrup is associated with increased pancreatic cancer risk" Aune D, Chan DSM, Vieira AR, et al. Dietary fructose, carbohydrates, glycemic indices and pancreatic cancer risk: a systemic review and meta-analysis of cohort studies. *Ann Oncol.* 2012;23(10):2536-2546.

Here are the most dangerous additives that you should remove from your diet as soon as you can:

1. Sugar, flour, enriched white flour, white flour, enriched bleached flour, enriched wheat flour, wheat flour, semolina flour, white rice, maltodextrin, glucose, high fructose corn syrup (HFCS), sucrose (table sugar), dextrose (corn sugar), and levulose

2. Artificial Sweeteners - listed as Sucralose, Aspartame, Acesulfame K, and Saccharin

3. Trans Fats and Partially Hydrogenated oils

4. MSG (also labeled as monosodium glutamate)

5. Excess Salt/Sodium in chips, crackers, canned food items, pickles, pretzels, condiments, and salted and sweetened nuts.

The choices are yours to make after you finish reading this book, as you are the only ONE who decides what to put in your digestive system!

Chapter 4

How to Alkalize your Body and KEEP it that way

The **best** and the **quickest way** you can **alkalize** your body and then maintain the degree of alkalinity your body requires to be most effective at neutralizing cancer cells will be for you to make the life sustaining decision to always make a point to only eat the foods your body's tissues and cells will require to keep you cancer free as well as lots of other major diseases. In reality this means you will consistently eat, on a daily basis, fresh, preferably organic vegetables, fruits and other foods that contain plenty of **cancer cell destroying properties of the alkalizing minerals** and **antioxidant vitamins found naturally within these foods which we examined in some detail in the chapter above.**

I also recommend that your decision to go alkaline include your beverages and that you make a point to drink alkalizing fresh fruit & vegetable juices that you can get at your local health or grocery store. The regular consumption of these kinds of juices, many of which are quite delicious – and others that will grow on you (no pun intended!) will further reduce the time it takes you to reach and maintain the level of alkalinity your body needs to avoid and defeat cancer.

Before we take a detailed look at the additional alkalizing food charts and tables later in the chapter which will guide you in what to select for your every day alkalizing nutrients and minerals, I want to stay on the subject of alkalizing beverages and introduce to you a **SUPER ALKALINE juice or pill supplement** which you may have heard of and which is commonly **known as "Wheatgrass".** I can't emphasize enough to you how beneficial this juice is to our bodies and therefore a juice that you should search out a local source for yourself immediately and then take it on a daily basis, preferably via **shots of fresh wheatgrass juice** on its own, as a friend of mine does, or mixed into a cocktail your fruit juice choices according to your taste preferences which is my personal preference.

Next, I go into detail with you about the benefits of this important juice which I make a point to take every day when there is an emergency and 2-3 times a week for a good benefit of your health. Investing in it now will cut dramatically your medical bills in the future!

WHEATGRASS IS ONE OF THE BEST ALKALINITY SOURCES FOR OUR BODIES

*"When we **love**, we always strive to become **better** than we are. When we strive **to become better** than we are, everything around us **becomes better too**."*

Paulo Coelho, the Alchemist

WHEATGRASS JUICE...

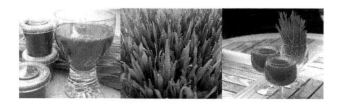

Wheatgrass should be recognized as very important for your body as it has the amazing ability to cleanse the blood, organs and gastrointestinal tract of **debris** and **toxins**; it **increases the red blood-cell count** and it also lowers blood pressure! Wheatgrass also stimulates your **metabolism** and the body's **enzyme systems** by enriching the blood. It aids in reducing blood pressure by dilating the blood pathways throughout the body.

Wheatgrass fights tumors and neutralizes toxins.

Recent studies show that wheatgrass juice has a powerful ability to **fight tumors** without the usual toxicity of drugs that also inhibit cell-destroying agents. The many active compounds found in wheatgrass juice cleanse the blood and neutralize and digest toxins in our cells.

As you know, chemotherapy and radiation treatments - as well as killing cancer cells - produce a lot of toxins, and a course of chemotherapy can destroy a lot of healthy cells. This is where **wheatgrass** comes as a hugely powerful **rejuvenating** and detoxifying tool.

The enzymes and amino acids found in wheatgrass can protect us from carcinogens like no other food or medicine. **It strengthens our cells**, **detoxifies** the **liver** and bloodstream, and chemically neutralizes environmental pollutants.

Wheatgrass juice also restores alkalinity to the blood. The juice's abundance of **alkaline minerals** helps **reduce over-acidity** in the blood. It can be used to relieve many internal pains, and has been used successfully to treat peptic ulcers, ulcerative colitis, constipation, diarrhea, and other complaints of the gastrointestinal tract.

Wheatgrass is a **concentrated** source of many nutrients, especially **Beta-carotene (Vitamin A), Calcium, Iron, Vitamin K, Vitamin C, Vitamin B12, Folic acid, Vitamin B6** and other trace nutrients.

Perhaps the reason this juice works so well for the human body is that Wheatgrass has a remarkable structural similarity to our own blood. Wheatgrass Juice is one of the best sources of **living chlorophyll available**. It contains **70% chlorophyll,** chlorophyll being the basis of all plant life.

Science has proven that chlorophyll **arrests growth** and **development** of unfriendly bacteria and helps to destroy **free radicals. Chlorophyll (wheatgrass juice)** has a nearly identical chemical structure to **hemoglobin (red blood cells),** which is the body's **critical oxygen** and **iron-carrying** blood protein. **Dr. Birscher**, a research scientist, called chlorophyll **"Concentrated Sun Power."** He says chlorophyll **increases** function of the **heart,** affects the **vascular system**, the **uterus**, the **intestine** and the **lungs**.

According to **Dr. Birscher**, nature uses chlorophyll as a **body cleanser**, **rebuilder** and **neutralizer of toxins**.

Dr. Yoshihide Hagiwara, president of the Hagiwara Institute of Health in Japan, is a leading advocate for the use of wheatgrass as **food** and **medicine**. He reasons that since chlorophyll is soluble in fat particles, and fat particles are absorbed directly into the blood via the lymphatic system, that chlorophyll can also be absorbed in this way. In other words, when the "blood" of plants is absorbed in humans it is transformed into human blood, which transports nutrients to **every cell of the body**.

Wheatgrass offers the benefits of a liquid oxygen transfusion since the juice contains liquid oxygen. **Oxygen** is vital to many body processes: it stimulates **digestion** (the oxidation of food), promotes **clearer thinking** (the brain utilizes 25% of the body's oxygen supply), and protects the blood against anaerobic bacteria. **Cancer cells cannot exist in the presence of oxygen**.

Interestingly, Wheatgrass has been found to turn grey hair to its natural color again and greatly increases energy levels, when consumed daily.

Please do not cook it! We can only get the benefits of the many enzymes found in wheatgrass by eating it fresh and uncooked. Cooking destroys **100 percent** of the **enzymes** that are so vital for us in food.

Wheatgrass can also:

- **Neutralize toxic substances** like cadmium, nicotine, strontium, mercury, and polyvinyl chloride.

- **Lessen the effects of radiation**. One enzyme found in wheatgrass, SOD, lessens the effects of radiation and acts as an anti-inflammatory compound that may **prevent cellular damage** following **heart attacks** or exposure to irritants.

Detoxification is the process of reducing the **"body burden"** by **eliminating toxins** that have been building for years or even decades. Because of the presence of **chlorophyll,** wheatgrass juice will cause detoxification to take place. If your body has stored toxins, it will Detox your body.

If you Detox too quickly, it is possible to have side effects that cause you to **temporarily** feel worse. When toxins re-enter the bloodstream, they can trigger an immune response that is termed a "healing crisis". This is a natural process, but can be uncomfortable and may include symptoms such as a headache (particularly for high sugar consumers, which I am sure you are avoiding now), flu-like feelings, diarrhea or fatigue. Start with a small amount of juice and work your way up to avoid this experience. It is necessary to drink plenty of water when detoxing, approximately 2 - 2.5 L a day. It's also very important not to drink any cold water or other drinks with meals; you should stop drinking water 15 min before a meal and start drinking 40-45 min after a meal (due to the quality of digestion). If Detox is noticeable, recognize it as a positive sign, consider reducing your juice consumption temporarily and be confident that it will pass. In a short period of time (1 day for some, less than 1 week for most, 1 month in rare circumstances) your body will be cleansed and you will experience the **mental**

clarity and physical **rejuvenation** that comes with **wheatgrass juice.**

As you can see, fresh wheatgrass juice (or any form available) will help you enormously to cope with chemotherapy side effects by **neutralizing chemicals** and **toxins**, increasing your **red blood cell** count, fighting with **tumors**, providing more **oxygen** to the cells and to the brain. All this is very critical and necessary help that you can provide for your body right now.

Suggested Dosage:

For normal health maintenance -1 to 4 oz. daily;
For therapeutic dosage - 4 to 8 oz. daily;
In cancer crisis - 10 oz. daily.

Wheatgrass is a powerful detoxifier of both the liver and large intestine. Ideally, people should gradually increase their intake from **one ounce** a day up to four to **eight ounces** spread throughout the day.

Recommended duration of an intake over four ounces a day is 60 days following which a "maintenance" level of two ounces a day intake will be most satisfactory.

The juice is taken on an empty stomach, at least 15 minutes before a meal.

JUICING OPTION

*"To **improve** is to **change**; to **be perfect** is **to change often.**"*

Winston Churchill

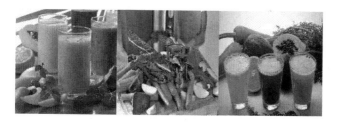

I want you to enjoy your more alkaline food and beverage diet every day, so here are several of my favorite combinations of the Super Alkaline Fresh Vegetables and Fresh Fruit Juices for you to enjoy and which will rebuild your body's natural defensive capabilities:

You do not actually have to go to a juice bar – you can also start making and drinking **fresh juices from organic fruits and vegetables** in your own kitchen and play with the ingredients according to your **own taste preferences**. I can give you a few ideas for **fresh juice** recipes and then you can involve your own creativity and imagination and create your own recipes knowing which vegetables and fruits to use from the charts in my book.

Sample these Delicious Fresh Vegetable Juice mixes – try to confirm from **organic sources**. You can decide the quantities of vegetables and fruits according to your own taste.

1. Apple

Carrot
Celery
Ginger
Spinach
Chia Seeds (or as a powder to have the best   absorption)
Fresh Wheatgrass - SUPER ALKALINE
(You can use wheatgrass powder or order frozen wheatgrass
if fresh wheatgrass juice is not accessible.)

2. Kale
   Cucumber
   Garlic
   Alfalfa
   Celeriac
   Chia Seeds as a powder
   Fresh Wheatgrass - SUPER ALKALINE

3. Apple - chew the seeds
   Pumpkin
   Spirulina
   Ginseng
   Chia Seeds as a powder
   Fresh Wheatgrass - SUPER ALKALINE

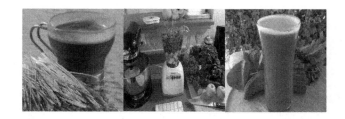

4. Alfalfa grass
   Spirulina
   Brussels sprouts
   Broccoli
   Chia Seeds as a powder
   Fresh Wheatgrass - SUPER ALKALINE

5. Kale
   Carrots
   Apricot seeds (kernels) – 2-3 pieces
   Alfalfa
   Bamboo
   Chia Seeds as a powder
   Fresh Wheatgrass - SUPER ALKALINE

Please experiment with the ingredients and quantities to find the combination that you like! You have to enjoy the taste. Please feel free to play with quantities according to your personal taste and preferences. Don't be put off by the color of some of these juice mixes, even the unappetizing colored juices can taste very delicious.

Now let's look at a few fresh **fruits - organic sources**:

1. Papaya
   Mango
   Lime
   Blackberries
   Chia Seeds as a powder
   Fresh Wheatgrass - SUPER ALKALINE

2. Banana
   Papaya

Coconut
Apple
Chia Seeds as a powder
Fresh Wheatgrass - SUPER ALKALINE

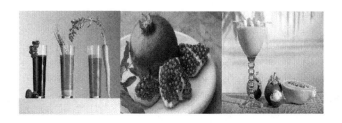

3. Pomegranate
Mango
Cranberry
Papaya
Chia Seeds as a powder
Fresh Wheatgrass - SUPER ALKALINE

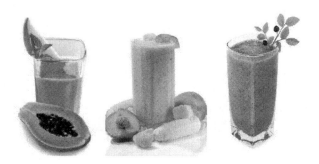

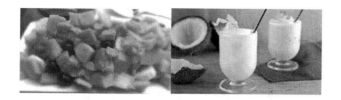

Based on the knowledge you've already learned above let's build on your understanding of the **solutions and actions you can confidently take now** if your saliva test is showing too much acidity.

As I explained earlier in the book, the first and most important step is to get your system **alkalized as quickly as possible** and you can start doing it today! Apart from adding **wheatgrass juice** and **chia seeds** to your daily diet, you should start using every day the charts in this book for reference, eating **organic** vegetables, fruits, beans, peas, whole grains, seeds and nuts, which are so full of **alkalizing minerals** and **antioxidant vitamins** as well as **cancer preventative enzymes**.

Now some details on Mother Nature's Super Antioxidant

We have available from Mother Nature another **Super Antioxidant**: **"Chia Seeds"** that I would like you to consider adding as a second daily dietary supplement along with your wheatgrass juice shots:

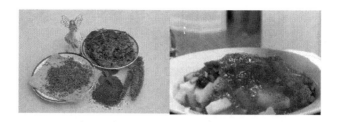

Chia is an astonishingly powerful **natural seed**. In 2008, a study by the Department of Foods and Nutrition, Purdue University, Indiana, USA reported that Chia contained, among other things, **significant amounts of antioxidants**.

Chia's army of antioxidants include flavonol aglycones: quercetin, kaempferol, and myricetin; and flavonol glycosides: **chlorogenic acid** and **caffeic acid.** These antioxidants have significant value to **human health.**

There are also reports saying that the **black Chia seeds** may contain 12%-15% more antioxidants that the **white seeds**. A study by the US-based Nutritional Science Research Institute performed a study on Chia seeds.

"... Chia seeds as one of the most powerful, whole food antioxidant we know."

Antioxidants contained in Chia seeds

Quercetin, one of Chia's **powerful antioxidants**, has been at the top of recent health news. Early this year, a study by researchers at the University of South Carolina's Arnold School of Public Health shows that *quercetin* significantly boosted energy, endurance and fitness in healthy men and women who were not involved in some type of daily physical training. This means that this antioxidant's fatigue-fighting properties could help average adults who battle fatigue and stress daily.

Quercetin, kaempferol, and *myricetin* are **antioxidants** that could protect against a host of chronic diseases like **ischemic heart disease**, cerebrovascular disease, **lung cancer**, **prostate cancer**, asthma, and **diabetes**.

Chlorogenic Acid, another of Chia's **antioxidants**, has been found by a study to possess **anti-cancer properties** and could be used to prevent growth of certain **brain tumors**. It could also slow the release of glucose into the bloodstream after a meal, and is a compound of interest for reducing the risk of developing Type 2 Diabetes. *Chlorogenic acids* do other things too: help the flow of bile, thus reducing bile stagnation and promoting **liver** and **gallbladder health**. It could also help to reduce cardiovascular risks. The body easily absorbs its nutritional benefits if it is sourced from natural, whole foods.

Caffeic acid, another antioxidant in Chia, may be used as a component to contribute to the prevention of the following: colitis, a condition that could lead to colon cancer, cardiovascular disease, **certain cancers,** mitosis (cell division) and inflammation. It may also be used in the healthy maintenance of the **immune system.**

Antioxidants in Chia seeds and oil help prevent cancer:

The most important antioxidants contained in Chia seeds are **chlorgenic acid** and **caffeic acid.** These are antioxidants that play a major role in **cancer prevention** and fighting **free radicals**.

Omega-3s

Chia seeds are the highest plant source of omega-3s. Omega-3s are healthy fatty acids that are needed for normal body and **brain functioning**, hormonal balance and the **absorption** of essential vitamins. Chia seeds consist of approximately 60 to 65 percent omega-3s, making them a potent **anti-inflammatory food**. Furthermore, since Chia seeds are a whole food and rich in antioxidants, they maintain freshness longer than most other sources of omega-3s such as fish oils and hemp seeds.

Recommended Doses:

Chia seeds are unique in that there is no recommended dosage or evidence of risks from possibly eating too much. The amount used varies among individuals, how they feel and their needs. Adults consuming Chia for general nutrition and health purposes, such as increased energy, might typically consume 2 tbsp. per day. I like to sprinkle ground chia seeds on my oat porridge in the morning.

100 grams (3.5oz.) of Omega^3 Chia is:

- a source of **Magnesium** equivalent to 53 ounces of Broccoli

- a source of **Iron** equivalent to 10 ounces of Spinach

- a source of **Folate** equivalent to 2 ounces of Asparagus

- a source of **Fiber** equivalent to 4 ounces of Bran

- a source of **Calcium** equivalent to 23 ounces of sesame seed

- a source of **Potassium** equivalent to 6 ounces of Bananas

- a source of **Antioxidants** equivalent to 10 ounces of Blueberries

- a source of **Omega3** Fatty Acids equivalent to 28 ounces of Atlantic Salmon

The above information shows you how rich Chia Seeds are in **alkalizing minerals** and full of **antioxidants** that can play a crucial role for you at this particular moment when you decided to get healthier, helping to quickly provide an alkalizing effect for your system. Chia seeds will also be important generally in the future to help you to continue staying healthy.

More about Antioxidants

Many foods, particularly those of the cabbage family, are found to increase **glutathione** levels in the body. **Selenium** and **glutathione** work together to protect fatty tissues such as **breast, liver** and **prostate. Glutathione** protects and regulates the **p53 tumour suppression gene** that could potentially prevent **half of all cancers. Bioflavonoids** are provided by green/blue/purple coloured foods (fruits, vegetables, berries, beans, spices, etc.). **Carotenoids** come from yellow/orange/red coloured foods. Many individual bioflavonoids and carotenoids have been shown to **inhibit**

cancer growth, and when you eat a variety of foods containing bioflavonoids and carotenoids, they work together to produce a very powerful effect on cancer.

Other antioxidants and antioxidant sources include resveratrol (found in grape skins), propolis, zinc, green tea, turmeric, L-carnosine, and organic germanium. Prunes also contain a very high concentration of antioxidants.

Now lets take a close look at vegetable oils.
Oxidized oils produce masses of free radicals in your body.
Vegetable oils (and margarine, made from these oils) are oils extracted from seeds like the rapeseed (canola oil) soybean (soybean oil), corn, sunflower, safflower, etc. They were practically non-existent in our diets until the early 1900s when new chemical processes allowed them to be extracted.
Here's the thing: Oxidized (rancid) vegetable oils like corn oil, soy oil, soybean oil, canola oil, sunflower oil etc., **break down under heat**, look the same as non-oxidized vegetable oils, but the **oxidized oils produce masses of free radicals in your body**.

The fat content of the human body is about 97% saturated and monounsaturated fat, with only 3 % Polyunsaturated fats. Half of that three percent is Omega-3 fats, and that balance needs to be there. Vegetable oils contain very high levels of polyunsaturated fats, and these oils have replaced many of the saturated fats in our diets since the 1950s.

The problem is that polyunsaturated fats are highly unstable and **oxidize** easily in the body if they haven't already oxidized during processing. **These oxidized fats cause inflammation and mutation in cells.**

In one study performed at the University of Western Ontario, researchers observed the effects of ten different dietary fats ranging from most saturated to least saturated. What they found is that saturated fats produced the least number of cancers, while omega-6 polyunsaturated fats produced the most. Numerous other studies have also shown that polyunsaturated fats stimulate cancer while saturated fat does not and that saturated fats do not break down to form free radicals.

Blaming saturated fat for heart disease "is the greatest biomedical error of the twentieth century."

Dr George Mann in the forward of Fat: "It's Not What You Think"

Refined, mostly polyunsaturated, vegetable oils have few, if any, available nutrients and are actually oxidized, or rancid, and add free radicals to the body. They're unstable when heated, cooking usually requires heating - forming additional free radicals.

Healthy cooking oils are natural and whole foods complete with a nutritional profile (i.e. containing bio-available nutrients) are a product of nature, not the laboratory, are stable when heated, and have a long tradition of use by healthy populations. Plant sources of saturated fat also do not convert into cholesterol.

This is the reason why I recommend that going forward you replace all vegetable cooking oils with either **coconut oil** or **extra virgin olive oil**.

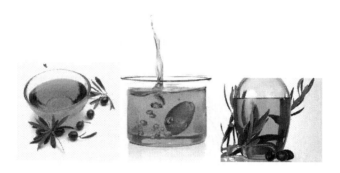

For good health, be sure to eat at least 3 or 4 tablespoons of coconut oil every day if possible. Start with teaspoon amounts and work up. **Coconut oil** is very easy to digest and provides an ideal source of energy for sick people and healthy people.

For general DNA repair in your body, it is also useful for your diet to include foods containing abundant nucleotides that are the building blocks from which your body builds DNA and RNA.

Foods providing nucleotides:
Sardines
Brewer's yeast
Anchovies
Mackerel
Lentils
Most beans
Chlorella algae
Spirulina algae.

Please note that in addition to providing your body with a steady supply of nucleotides, removing excess **acidity** from the system and maintaining lower alkalinity will allow your body tissues to become aerobic and be responsive to the **DNA self-repair mechanism that can only function when alkalinity levels are normal.**

Essential Amino Acids

Amino acids are described as the "building blocks of protein," and they are important to the synthesis of proteins and the **overall functioning of the body**. In particular, there are 10 amino acids classified as **"essential,"** which means they are not naturally made by the human body. These amino acids must be acquired through the foods you eat, reports the University of Arizona Department of Biochemistry, or your body will begin to break down existing protein, such as **muscle tissue**. Unlike fat, amino acids can't be stored in the body for later use. Therefore, it is doubly important that you include these amino acids in your diet on a consistent basis.

Nuts

Nuts and **legumes** are abundant sources of amino acids. Walnuts, almonds, Brazil nuts, cashews and peanuts are all rich sources of the essential amino acid L-arginine. Arginine is known to **boost immune function**, assist in **muscle metabolism** and muscle mass and enhance collagen production and bone growth. Almonds and cashews are also top sources of isoleucine, another essential amino acid that stabilizes blood sugar and increases energy. Almonds and peanuts also boast high levels of the amino acid phenylalanine, which is thought to enhance mood.

Wild Fish

Wild fish of any kind is another top source of many of the amino acids. Fatty fish such as salmon, tuna, herring and sardines are also rich in omega-3 fatty acids, which may have benefits in protecting against heart disease. Fish are abundant in the essential amino acids isoleucine, lysine and methionine.

Free-range eggs

Free-range eggs contain plentiful amounts of amino acids and are an excellent source of protein for relatively few calories. Eggs are good sources of the essential amino acids methionine, isoleucine and lysine. They are a good source of tryptophan, an essential amino acid involved in the production of the mood-enhancing neurotransmitter serotonin.

Whole eggs provide your body with a source of fat-soluble vitamins, including A, D and E, significant quantities of certain B complex vitamins, including B-6, B-12, folate and riboflavin and alkaline minerals such as **calcium, magnesium**, iron, zinc and **selenium**. As well as everything else you should eat them in moderation.

As I promised to you earlier in the book that you will enjoy your food, I thought I would give you a few more ideas for cooking food that is good for your body. You will have even more interesting and creative ideas yourself and create your own favorite recipes.

Roasted Chickpeas

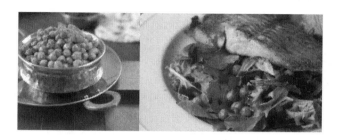

Ingredients:

3/4 tsp Cumin seeds
3/4 tsp Coriander seeds
350 g Cooked chickpeas, drained
1 tbsp Extra-virgin olive oil
Pinch of cayenne pepper
Sea salt

Method:

Preheat oven to 200C/400F. Toast cumin seeds and coriander seeds in small skillet over medium heat until beginning to brown, about 2 minutes. Cool. Transfer to spice mill and process until finely ground.

Place chickpeas, olive oil, pinch of cayenne, and ground spices in medium bowl. Sprinkle with salt, then toss to coat evenly. Transfer to small-rimmed baking sheet. Roast in oven until lightly browned and crunchy, stirring occasionally, about 35 minutes.

Can be made 4 hours ahead. Let stand at room temperature. Reheat in 200C/400F oven until warm, about 5 minutes, before serving.

Whole wheat Penne with Arugula and Avocado

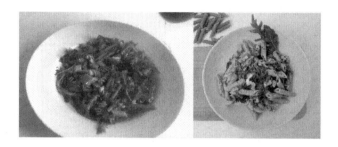

Ingredients:

200 g Whole wheat penne
3 cup Baby arugula leaves
3-5 Garlic cloves, sliced
40 g Walnuts, toasted
One Avocado
70 ml Olive oil
Sea salt and freshly ground pepper

Method:

Bring a large pot of water to a rapid boil. Add 1 teaspoon of sea salt and the pasta to the boiling water and stir. Boil gently uncovered, stirring occasionally. Follow package directions and cook until al dente stage, chewy but not hard.

Meanwhile, combine arugula, garlic slices, walnuts in a food processor. With the machine running, slowly drizzle in olive oil and process until evenly blended. Season pesto well with sea salt and freshly ground black pepper. Mix until evenly combined.

Drain pasta and return to the pot. Add arugula pesto and sliced avocado and toss well. Serve immediately. The pesto will keep about 1 week in a tightly sealed container in the refrigerator.

Quinoa cookies with Rye Flakes and Flaxseed

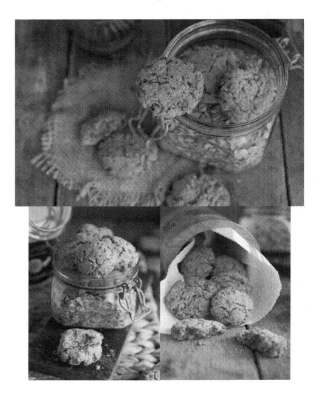

These cookies are made using **nutrient-dense quinoa**, a complete protein, rich in **iron**, **minerals** and **amino acids**, **rye flakes** and **flaxseed**. You can experiment by replacing rye flakes with oats or quinoa flakes or a mix of two. Dark chocolate chips can also be added for a richer, moister taste. And of course you can always frost them with dark chocolate. Enjoy them as a wholesome breakfast or as a tasty snack any time you like.

150 g Rye flakes
150 g Cooked quinoa
2 tbsp Flaxseed
70 g Brown sugar
2 tbsp Vanilla protein powder
½ tsp Baking soda
2 tsp Baking powder
90 ml Coconut oil, melted
70 ml Maple syrup
1 tsp Vanilla extract
2-3 tbsp Coconut milk

- Melt the coconut oil over low heat. Set aside to cool. Roughly blend rye flakes into powder. Preheat the oven to 180C/350F.
- Whisk together the blended rye flakes, cooked quinoa, flaxseed, brown sugar, vanilla protein powder, baking soda, and baking powder in a large mixing bowl.

Stir in melted coconut oil, maple syrup, vanilla extract and coconut milk. Mix to combine. Shape the dough into inch balls and flatten each into a round circle with the palm of your hand. Place them on the parchment-lined baking trays. Bake for 10 minutes until golden brown.

Now you can improvise so much with different grains and

your favorite vegetables and nuts. I would now like you to take a close look at the Nuts chart presenting the amount of mineral and vitamins as well as complete protein in nuts, seeds and whole grains all of which will help you create delicious meals. To add more variety to your alkaline food selections, you will want to frequently include nuts, seed and grains that you like into your meals.

A lot of people are worried about eating nuts as they are concerned about fat. Fortunately, in the case of nuts, they contain "good" fats as discussed below.

Good healthy fat is the most important macronutrient, as it is needed to make **every cell** and **every hormone**. **Good fats** are also used to keep the hair and skin healthy, maintain proper **inflammation function**, and keep our **moods stable**.

Good fats are called essential fatty acids (EFAs) and are found in food such as **fish and shellfish, flaxseed, hemp oil, olive oil, chia seeds, pumpkin seeds, sunflower seeds, leafy vegetables, and nuts.** We need an abundance of good fats in our diets because the **body cannot make these "essential" fatty acids.**

Eating these good fats uncouples or breaks apart the **stored body fat** so it can be burned for fuel easier, as a result making us **leaner**. Try adding more **good fat** to your diet and you will be amazed at how **good you look and feel**!
And studies have found that foods with good healthy fats, like **avocado** and **nuts**, take longer to digest and therefore help keep you fuller longer. Nuts, seeds and grains also providing us with alkalizing minerals as well as with some

antioxidant vitamins as you see in the chart below.

Best Alkalizing Nuts, Seeds and Grains chart with Mineral and Vitamin content

Nut/Seed	Protein/Fiber	Minerals	Vitamins
Almonds	1 ounce (23 whole nuts) of raw almonds contains 6.02 grams protein, 163 calories and 3.5 grams of dietary fiber.	Potassium - 200 mg Phosphorus - 137 mg Calcium - 75 mg Magnesium - 76 mg Iron - 1.05 mg Selenium - 0.7 mcg Zinc - 0.87 mg Manganese - 0.648 mg Copper - 0.282 mg Also contains a small amount of other minerals.	Vitamin B1 (thiamine) - 0.06 mg Vitamin B2 (riboflavin) - 0.287 mg Niacin - 0.96 mg Folate - 14 mcg Pantothenic Acid - 0.133 mg Vitamin B6 - 0.041 mg Vitamin E - 7.43 mg Contains some other vitamins in small amounts.
Amaranth	100 grams of cooked amaranth contain 3.8 grams protein, 102 calories and 2.1 grams dietary fiber.	Potassium - 135 mg Phosphorus - 148 mg Calcium - 47 mg Magnesium - 65 mg Iron - 2.1 mg Sodium - 6 mg Manganese - 0.854 mg Zinc - 0.86 mg Copper - 0.149 mg Selenium - 5.5 mcg Also contains trace amounts of other minerals.	Vitamin B1 (thiamine) - 0.015 mg Vitamin B2 (riboflavin) - 0.022 mg Niacin - 0.235 mg Vitamin B6 - 0.113 mg Folate - 22 mcg Vitamin E - 0.19 mg Contains some other vitamins in small amounts.
Barley (Pearled)	100 grams of cooked, pearled barley contain 2.26 grams	Potassium - 93 mg Phosphorus - 54 mg Calcium - 11 mg Magnesium - 22	Vitamin B1 (thiamine) - 0.083 mg Vitamin B2 (riboflavin) - 0.062 mg

	protein, 123 calories and 3.8 grams dietary fiber.	mg Iron - 1.33 mg Sodium - 3 mg Manganese - 0.259 mg Zinc - 0.82 mg Copper - 0.105 mg Selenium - 8.6 mcg Also contains trace amounts of other minerals.	Niacin - 2.063 mg Pantothenic Acid - 0.135 mg Vitamin B6 - 0.115 mg Folate - 16 mcg Vitamin A - 7 IU Vitamin E - 0.01 mg Vitamin K - 0.8 mcg Contains some other vitamins in small amounts.
Brazil Nuts 	1 ounce (6 whole nuts) contains 4.06 grams of protein, 186 calories and 2.1 grams of fiber.	Potassium - 187 mg Phosphorus - 206 mg Calcium - 45 mg Magnesium - 107 mg Iron - 0.69 mg Sodium - 1 mg Manganese - 0.347 mg Zinc - 1.15 mg Copper - 0.494 mg Selenium - 543.5 mcg Also contains trace amounts of other minerals.	Vitamin C - 0.2 mg Vitamin B1 (thiamine) - 0.175 mg Vitamin B2 (riboflavin) - 0.01 mg Niacin - 0.084 mg Pantothenic Acid - 0.052 mg Vitamin B6 - 0.029 mg Folate - 6 mcg Vitamin E - 1.62 mg Contains some other vitamins in small amounts.
Buckwheat 	100 grams of buckwheat contain 13.25 grams protein, 343 calories and 10 grams dietary fiber.	Potassium - 460 mg Phosphorus - 347 mg Calcium - 18 mg Magnesium - 231 mg Iron - 2.2 mg Sodium - 1 mg Manganese - 1.3 mg Zinc - 2.4 mg Copper - 1.1 mg Selenium - 8.3 mcg Also contains trace amounts of other minerals.	Vitamin B1 (thiamine) - 0.101 mg Vitamin B2 (riboflavin) - 0.425 mg Niacin - 7.02 mg Pantothenic Acid - 1.233 mg Vitamin B6 - 0.21 mg Folate - 30 mcg Contains some other vitamins in small amounts.
Cashews	One ounce of raw, unsalted cashew nuts contains 5.17 grams of protein, 157	Potassium - 187 mg Phosphorus - 168 mg Calcium - 10 mg Magnesium - 83	Vitamin C - 0.1 mg Vitamin B1 (thiamine) - 0.12 mg Vitamin B2 (riboflavin) - 0.016

	calories and 0.94 grams of fiber.	mg Iron - 1.89 mg Sodium - 3 mg Manganese - 0.469 mg Zinc - 1.64 mg Copper - 0.622 mg Selenium - 5.6 mcg Also contains trace amounts of other minerals.	mg Niacin - 0.301 mg Pantothenic Acid - 0.245 mg Vitamin B6 - 0.118 mg Folate - 7 mcg Vitamin E - 0.26 mg Vitamin K - 9.7 mcg Contains some other vitamins in small amounts.
Chestnuts	Ten (10) roasted kernels with no salt added contain 2.66 grams protein, 206 calories and 4.3 grams fiber. (Note: chestnuts must be boiled or roasted before eating due to the high levels of tannic acid.)	Potassium - 497 mg Phosphorus - 90 mg Calcium - 24 mg Magnesium - 28 mg Iron - 0.76 mg Sodium - 2 mg Manganese - 0.991 mg Zinc - 0.48 mg Copper - 0.426 mg Selenium - 1 mcg Also contains trace amounts of other minerals.	Vitamin C - 21.8 mg Vitamin B1 (thiamine) - 0.204 mg Vitamin B2 (riboflavin) - 0.147 mg Niacin - 1.127 mg Pantothenic Acid - 0.465 mg Vitamin B6 - 0.417 mg Folate - 59 mcg Vitamin A - 20 IU Vitamin E - 0.42 mg Vitamin K - 6.6 mcg Contains some other vitamins in small amounts.
Coconut	One cup of raw, shredded coconut contains 2.66 grams of protein, 283 calories and 7.2 grams of dietary fiber.	Potassium - 285 mg Phosphorus - 90 mg Calcium - 11 mg Magnesium - 26 mg Iron - 1.94 mg Sodium - 16 mg Manganese - 1.2 mg Zinc - 0.88 mg Copper - 0.348 mg Selenium - 8.1 mcg Also contains trace amounts of other minerals.	Vitamin C - 2.6 mg Vitamin B1 (thiamine) - 0.053 mg Vitamin B2 (riboflavin) - 0.016 mg Niacin - 0.432 mg Pantothenic Acid - 0.24 mg Vitamin B6 - 0.043 mg Folate - 21 mcg Vitamin E - 0.19 mg Vitamin K - 0.2 mcg Contains some other vitamins in small amounts.
Flax Seed	One tablespoon of raw flax	Potassium - 84 mg Phosphorus - 66	Vitamin C 0.1 mg Vitamin B1 (thiamine) - 0.169

	seeds contains 1.88 grams of protein, 55 calories and 2.8 grams of dietary fiber.	mg Calcium - 26 mg Magnesium - 40 mg Iron - 0.59 mg Sodium - 3 mg Manganese - 0.256 mg Zinc - 0.45 mg Copper - 0.126 mg Selenium - 2.6 mcg Also contains trace amounts of other minerals.	mg Vitamin B2 (riboflavin) - 0.017 mg Niacin - 0.317 mg Pantothenic Acid - 0.101 mg Vitamin B6 - 0.049 mg Folate - 9 mcg Vitamin E - 0.03 mg Vitamin K - 0.4 mcg Contains some other vitamins in small amounts.
Hazelnuts	One ounce (21 whole kernels) of hazelnuts contains 4.24 grams of protein, 178 calories and 2.7 grams of dietary fiber.	Potassium - 193 mg Phosphorus - 82 mg Calcium - 32 mg Magnesium - 46 mg Iron - 1.33 mg Manganese - 1.751 mg Zinc - 0.69 mg Copper - 0.489 mg Selenium - 0.7 mcg Also contains trace amounts of other minerals.	Vitamin C - 1.8 mg Vitamin B1 (thiamine) - 0.182 mg Vitamin B2 (riboflavin) - 0.032 mg Niacin - 0.51 mg Pantothenic Acid - 0.26 mg Vitamin B6 - 0.16 mg Folate - 32 mcg Vitamin A - 6 IU Vitamin E - 4.26 mg Vitamin K - 4 mcg Contains some other vitamins in small amounts.
Macadamias	One once (10-12 kernels) of raw macadamia nuts contains 2.24 grams protein, 204 calories and 2.4 grams fiber.	Potassium - 104 mg Phosphorus - 53 mg Calcium - 24 mg Magnesium - 37 mg Iron - 1.05 mg Sodium - 1 mg Manganese - 1.171 mg Zinc - 0.37 mg Copper - 0.214 mg Selenium - 1 mcg Also contains trace amounts of other minerals.	Vitamin C - 0.3 mg Vitamin B1 (thiamine) - 0.339 mg Vitamin B2 (riboflavin) - 0.046 mg Niacin - 0.701 mg Pantothenic Acid - 0.215 mg Vitamin B6 - 0.078 mg Folate - 3 mcg Vitamin E - 0.15 mg Contains some other vitamins in small amounts.
Millet	100 grams of	Potassium - 62	Vitamin B1

	cooked millet contain 3.51 grams protein, 119 calories and 1.3 grams dietary fiber.	mg Phosphorus - 100 mg Calcium - 3 mg Magnesium - 44 mg Iron - 0.63 mg Sodium - 2 mg Manganese - 0.272 mg Zinc - 0.91 mg Copper - 0.161 mg Selenium - 0.9 mcg Also contains trace amounts of other minerals.	(thiamine) - 0.106 mg Vitamin B2 (riboflavin) - 0.082 mg Niacin - 1.33 mg Pantothenic Acid - 0.171 mg Vitamin B6 - 0.108 mg Folate - 19 mcg Vitamin A - 3 IU Vitamin E - 0.02 mg Vitamin K - 0.3 mcg Contains some other vitamins in small amounts.
Oats	100 grams of oats contain grams 16.89 protein, 389 calories and 10.6 grams dietary fiber.	Potassium - 429 mg Phosphorus - 523 mg Calcium - 54 mg Magnesium - 177 mg Iron - 4.72 mg Sodium - 2 mg Manganese - 4.916 mg Zinc - 3.97 mg Copper - 0.626 mg Also contains trace amounts of other minerals.	Vitamin B1 (thiamine) - 0.763 mg Vitamin B2 (riboflavin) - 0.139 mg Niacin - 0.961 mg Pantothenic Acid - 1.349 mg Vitamin B6 - 0.119 mg Folate - 56 mcg Contains some other vitamins in small amounts.
Peanuts	One ounce of dry roasted peanuts contains 6.71 grams of protein, 166 calories and 2.3 grams of dietary fiber.	Potassium -187 mg Phosphorus - 101 mg Calcium - 15 mg Magnesium - 50 mg Iron - 0.64 mg Sodium - 2 mg Manganese - 0.591 mg Zinc - 0.94 mg Copper - 0.190 mg Selenium - 2.1 mcg Also contains trace amounts of other minerals.	Vitamin B1 (thiamine) - 0.124 mg Vitamin B2 (riboflavin) - 0.028 mg Niacin - 3.834 mg Pantothenic Acid - 0.395 mg Vitamin B6 - 0.073 mg Folate - 41 mcg Vitamin E - 1.96 mg Contains some other vitamins in small amounts.
Pecans	One ounce (19 halves) of	Potassium - 116 mg	Vitamin C - 0.3 mg Vitamin B1

	raw pecans contains 2.6 grams protein, 196 calories and 2.7 grams fiber.	Phosphorus - 79 mg Calcium - 20 mg Magnesium - 34 mg Iron - 0.72 mg Manganese - 1.276 mg Zinc - 1.28 mg Copper - 0.34 mg Selenium - 1.1 mcg Also contains trace amounts of other minerals.	(thiamine) - 0.187 mg Vitamin B2 (riboflavin) - 0.01 mg Niacin - 0.331 mg Pantothenic Acid - 0.245 mg Vitamin B6 - 0.06 mg Folate - 6 mcg Vitamin A - 16 IU Vitamin E - 0.4 mg Vitamin K - 1 mcg Contains some other vitamins in small amounts.
Pine Nuts / Pignolias 	One ounce of pine nuts (167 kernels) contains 3.88 grams of protein, 191 calories and 1.0 grams of dietary fiber.	Potassium - 169 mg Phosphorus - 163 mg Calcium - 5 mg Magnesium - 71 mg Iron - 1.57 mg Sodium - 1 mg Manganese - 2.495 mg Zinc - 1.83 mg Copper - 0.375 mg Selenium - 0.2 mcg Also contains trace amounts of other minerals.	Vitamin C - 0.2 mg Vitamin B1 (thiamine) - 0.103 mg Vitamin B2 (riboflavin) - 0.064 mg Niacin - 1.244 mg Pantothenic Acid - 0.089 mg Vitamin B6 - 0.027 mg Folate - 10 mcg Vitamin A - 8 IU Vitamin E - 2.65 mg Vitamin K - 15.3 mcg Contains some other vitamins in small amounts.
Pistachios 	One ounce of dry roasted pistachio nuts (no salt) (49 kernels) contains 6.05 grams of protein, 162 calories and 2.9 grams of dietary fiber.	Potassium - 295 mg Phosphorus - 137 mg Calcium - 31 mg Magnesium - 34 mg Iron - 1.19 mg Sodium - 3 mg Manganese - 0.361 mg Zinc - 0.65 mg Copper - 0.376 mg Selenium - 2.6 mcg Also contains trace amounts of other minerals.	Vitamin C - 0.7 mg Vitamin B1 (thiamine) - 0.238 mg Vitamin B2 (riboflavin) - 0.045 mg Niacin - 0.404 mg Pantothenic Acid - 0.145 mg Vitamin B6 - 0.361 mg Folate - 14 mcg Vitamin A - 74 IU Vitamin E - 0.55 mg Vitamin K - 3.7 mcg Contains some other vitamins in

			small amounts.
Pumpkin Seeds	One ounce of roasted pumpkin or squash seed kernels (no salt) contains 8.46 grams of protein, 163 calories and 1.8 grams of dietary fiber.	Potassium - 223 mg Phosphorus - 333 mg Calcium - 15 mg Magnesium - 156 mg Iron - 2.29 mg Sodium - 5 mg Manganese - 1.273 mg Zinc - 2.17 mg Copper - 0.361 mg Selenium - 2.7 mcg Also contains trace amounts of other minerals.	Vitamin C - 0.5 mg Vitamin B1 (thiamine) - 0.02 mg Vitamin B2 (riboflavin) - 0.043 mg Niacin - 1.256 mg Pantothenic Acid - 0.162 mg Vitamin B6 - 0.028 mg Folate - 16 mcg Vitamin A - 2 IU Vitamin E - 0.16 mg Vitamin K - 1.3 mcg Contains some other vitamins in small amounts.
Quinoa	100 grams of cooked quinoa contain 4.4 grams protein, 120 calories and 2.8 grams dietary fiber.	Potassium - 172 mg Phosphorus - 152 mg Calcium - 17 mg Magnesium - 64 mg Iron - 1.49 mg Sodium - 7 mg Manganese - 0.631 mg Zinc - 1.09 mg Copper - 0.192 mg Selenium - 2.8 mcg Also contains trace amounts of other minerals.	Vitamin B1 (thiamine) - 0.107 mg Vitamin B2 (riboflavin) - 0.11 mg Niacin - 0.412 mg Vitamin B6 - 0.123 mg Folate - 42 mcg Vitamin A - 5 IU Vitamin E - 0.63 mg Contains some other vitamins in small amounts.
Rice - Brown	100 grams of cooked brown rice contain 2.32 grams of protein, 112 calories and 1.8 grams of dietary fiber.	Potassium - 79 mg Phosphorus - 77 mg Calcium - 10 mg Magnesium - 44 mg Iron - 0.53 mg Sodium - 1 mg Manganese - 1.097 mg Zinc - 0.62 mg Copper - 0.081 mg Also contains trace amounts of	Vitamin B1 (thiamine) - 0.102 mg Vitamin B2 (riboflavin) - 0.012 mg Niacin - 1.33 mg Pantothenic Acid - 0.392 mg Vitamin B6 - 0.149 mg Folate - 4 mcg Contains some other vitamins in small amounts.

		other minerals.	
Rice - Wild	100 grams of cooked wild rice contain 3.99 grams of protein, 101 calories and 1.8 grams of dietary fiber	Potassium - 101 mg Phosphorus - 82 mg Calcium - 3 mg Magnesium - 32 mg Iron - 0.6 mg Sodium - 3 mg Manganese - 0.282 mg Zinc - 1.34 mg Copper - 0.121 mg Selenium - 0.8 mcg Also contains trace amounts of other minerals.	Vitamin B1 (thiamine) - 0.052 mg Vitamin B2 (riboflavin) - 0.087 mg Niacin - 1.287 mg Pantothenic Acid - 0.154 mg Vitamin B6 - 0.135 mg Folate - 26 mcg Vitamin A - 3 IU Vitamin E - 0.24 mg Vitamin K - 0.5 mcg Contains some other vitamins in small amounts.
Rye	100 grams of rye contain 10.34 grams protein, 338 calories and 14.6 grams dietary fiber.	Potassium - 510 mg Phosphorus - 332 mg Calcium - 24 mg Magnesium - 110 mg Iron - 2.63 mg Sodium - 2 mg Manganese - 2.577 mg Zinc - 2.65 mg Copper - 0.367 mg Selenium - 13.9 mcg Also contains trace amounts of other minerals.	Vitamin B1 (thiamine) - 0.316 mg Vitamin B2 (riboflavin) - 0.251 mg Niacin - 4.27 mg Pantothenic Acid - 1.456 mg Vitamin B6 - 0.294 mg Folate - 38 mcg Vitamin A - 11 IU Vitamin E - 0.85 mg Vitamin K - 5.9 mcg Contains some other vitamins in small amounts.
Sesame Seeds	One tablespoon of dried sesame seeds (no salt) contains 1.6 grams of protein, 52 calories and 1.1 grams of dietary fiber.	Potassium - 42 mg Phosphorus - 57 mg Calcium - 88 mg Magnesium - 32 mg Iron - 1.31 mg Sodium - 1 mg Manganese - 0.221 mg Zinc - 0.7 mg Copper - 0.367 mg Selenium - 3.1 mcg Also contains	Vitamin B1 (thiamine) - 0.071 mg Vitamin B2 (riboflavin) - 0.022 mg Niacin - 0.406 mg Pantothenic Acid - 0.005 mg Vitamin B6 - 0.071 mg Folate - 9 mcg Vitamin A - 1 IU Vitamin E - 0.02 mg Contains some other vitamins in

		trace amounts of other minerals.	small amounts.
Spelt	100 grams of cooked, spelt contain 5.5 grams protein, 127 calories and 3.9 grams dietary fiber.	Potassium - 143 mg Phosphorus - 150 mg Calcium - 10 mg Magnesium - 49 mg Iron - 1.67 mg Sodium - 5 mg Manganese - 1.091 mg Zinc - 1.25 mg Copper - 0.215 mg Selenium - 4 mcg Also contains trace amounts of other minerals.	Vitamin B1 (thiamine) - 0.103 mg Vitamin B2 (riboflavin) - 0.03 mg Niacin - 2.57 mg Vitamin B6 - 0.08 mg Folate - 13 mcg Vitamin A - 4 IU Vitamin E - 0.26 mg Contains some other vitamins in small amounts.
Sunflower Seeds	One ounce of sunflower seed kernels, dry-roasted without salt contains 5.48 grams of protein, 165 calories and 3.1 grams of dietary fiber.	Potassium - 241 mg Phosphorus - 327 mg Calcium - 20 mg Magnesium - 37 mg Iron - 1.08 mg Sodium - 1 mg Manganese - 0.598 mg Zinc - 1.5 mg Copper - 0.519 mg Selenium - 22.5 mcg Also contains trace amounts of other minerals.	Vitamin C - 0.4 mg Vitamin B1 (thiamine) - 0.03 mg Vitamin B2 (riboflavin) - 0.07 mg Niacin - 1.996 mg Pantothenic Acid - 1.996 mg Vitamin B6 - 0.228 mg Folate - 67 mcg Vitamin A - 3 IU Vitamin E - 7.4 mg Vitamin K - 0.8 mcg Contains some other vitamins in small amounts.
Walnuts	1 ounce (14 halves) English walnuts contain 4.32 mg protein, 185 calories and 1.9 mg fiber.	Potassium - 125 mg Phosphorus - 98 mg Calcium - 28 mg Magnesium - 45 mg Iron - 0.82 mg Sodium - 1 mg Manganese - 0.968 mg Zinc - 0.88 mg Copper - 0.45 mg Selenium - 1.4 mcg	Vitamin C - 0.4 mg Vitamin B1 (thiamine) - 0.097 mg Vitamin B2 (riboflavin) - 0.043 mg Niacin - 0.319 mg Pantothenic Acid - 0.162 mg Vitamin B6 - 0.152 mg Folate - 28 mcg Vitamin A - 6 IU Vitamin E - 0.2 mg Vitamin K - 0.8 mcg

		Also contains trace amounts of other minerals.	Contains some other vitamins in small amounts.
Wheat - Durum	100 grams of durum wheat contain 13.68 grams protein and 339 calories.	Potassium - 431 mg Phosphorus - 508 mg Calcium - 34 mg Magnesium - 144 mg Iron - 3.52 mg Sodium - 2 mg Manganese - 3.012 mg Zinc - 4.16 mg Copper - 0.553 mg Selenium - 89.4 mcg Also contains trace amounts of other minerals.	Vitamin B1 (thiamine) - 0.419 mg Vitamin B2 (riboflavin) - 0.121 mg Niacin - 6.738 mg Pantothenic Acid - 0.935 mg Vitamin B6 - 0.419 mg Folate - 43 mcg Contains some other vitamins in small amounts.
Wheat - Hard Red	100 grams of hard red wheat contain 15.40 grams protein, 329 calories and 12.2 grams of dietary fiber.	Potassium - 340 mg Phosphorus - 332 mg Calcium - 25 mg Magnesium - 124 mg Iron - 3.6 mg Sodium - 2 mg Manganese - 4.055 mg Zinc - 2.78 mg Copper - 0.41 mg Selenium - 70.7 mcg Also contains trace amounts of other minerals.	Vitamin B1 (thiamine) - 0.504 mg Vitamin B2 (riboflavin) - 0.11 mg Niacin - 5.71 mg Pantothenic Acid - 0.935 mg Vitamin B6 - 0.336 mg Folate - 43 mcg Vitamin A - 9 IU Vitamin E - 1.01 mg Vitamin K - 1.9 mcg Contains some other vitamins in small amounts.
Whole Wheat	100 grams of hard white wheat contain 11.31 grams protein, 342 calories and 12.2 grams dietary fiber.	Potassium - 432 mg Phosphorus - 355 mg Calcium - 32 mg Magnesium - 93 mg Iron - 4.56 mg Sodium - 2 mg Manganese - 3.821 mg Zinc - 3.33 mg Copper - 0.363 mg Also contains	Vitamin B1 (thiamine) - 0.387 mg Vitamin B2 (riboflavin) - 0.108 mg Niacin - 4.381 mg Pantothenic Acid - 0.954 mg Vitamin B6 - 0.368 mg Folate - 38 mcg Vitamin A - 9 IU Vitamin E - 1.01 mg

		trace amounts of other minerals.	Vitamin K - 1.9 mcg Contains some other vitamins in small amounts.

Chapter 5

"Acknowledging the good that you already have in your life is the foundation for all abundance."

Eckhart Tolle

How Free Radicals And Toxins Poison Cells

Every day our bodies and cells are under **attack** from **free radicals** and **toxins** from processed, high fat foods, stress, every day household chemicals, pollution, sun exposure, ozone. This causes the DNA inside cells to break down and lose their ability to make sharp "carbon copies".

Just as your body needs food to survive, your **cells need nutrition to live and healthily regenerate.** Here is the issue - what is the overall quality of food we are providing our bodies with on a day to day basis? A lot of foods people eat these days, such as processed foods, are nutrient-depleted foods, which puts our body cells in a **nutritionally starved mode**. When our body cells do not get essential life – giving Omega 3s, essential vitamins and minerals from natural food, powerful antioxidants and essential fatty acids (EFAs) they are literally being starved to death! **They slowly shrink and then die off**. If you are not currently flooding your cells with Life-Giving nutrients now, then you are wide open to accelerated disease and aging…This is not meant to scare you, just become aware that you are the only one responsible for your own quality of health and that you are more than able to make sure your body receives what it would choose for itself if it could make the decisions for you.

Unlike the health challenges of the past, which were predominantly due to infectious diseases, our modern health epidemics such as cardiovascular disease, diabetes, dementia, cancer, and obesity are fueled by a one-two punch of **chronic inflammation** within the body and extensive **free radical damage to our cells.**

The Challenge of Inflammation and Free Radical Damage

In the world of medicine, it is now accepted that **inflammation** and **free radical damage** are two of the **greatest threats** to our health.

Free radicals are the other great threat, causing a condition known as **oxidation**, or **oxidative stress**. In the material world oxidation is observed as **rust**; and a similar process occurs **within our bodies**. Dr. Ames, from the University of California, Berkeley believes, *"Free Radical Oxidant by-products of normal metabolism cause extensive damage to DNA, proteins, and lipids."* This damage is a major contributor to aging and to degenerative diseases such as

cancer, cardiovascular disease, immune system decline, brain dysfunction, and **cataracts**.

Oxidative stress and inflammation are intimately connected, each fueling the other. A vicious cycle is created: free radical damage leads to inflammation and inflammation causes free radical damage.

The key to recovering and preserving our health requires both the quenching of inflammation and the prevention of excessive free radical damage.

I would like you to see the **relationship** between **free radicals** and **cancer cells**. First of all lets understand the nature of free radicals. A **harmful free radical** is an **ion** that has a positive electrical charge. An electron has a negative electrical charge. Due to its positive charge, the free radical attracts electrons from other molecules, thereby damaging them. One of the causes of cancer is excessive free radical damage in your cells that harms your DNA and results in some cells **mutating** into cancerous cells.

Every chemical and toxin in your body causes free radical damage. The carcinogenic ones cause even more. Combined with high acidity and low oxygenation a lot of people get a prescription for cancer. Free radical damage from toxins plays a fundamental role in the development of cancer.

Sources of free radicals include farm chemicals (fertilizers and pesticides), many prescription drugs, processed foods, cigarette smoke, environmental pollution, alcohol, electromagnetic radiation, and stress. (Sharma, pages 26-27).

Antioxidants get rid of free radicals

You already learned a lot about the power of antioxidants in Chapter 2 and Chapter 3 and now I would like to introduce you a Super special antioxidant found in the sea!

Ecklonia Cava is a brown algae (seaweed) that grows off the coast of Japan and Korea proven **100 times more powerful than any land-based antioxidants**. Over 15 years of research and nearly 40 million USD worth of clinical studies back it up. It's the only **FDA-approved Ecklonia Cava marine algae** extract in existence. It works in your body for 12 hours compared to land based Antioxidants that work only for 30 minutes. *Ecklonia cava* is a potent antioxidant that has the ability to pass through the **blood-brain barrier**, which means it can reach the brain.

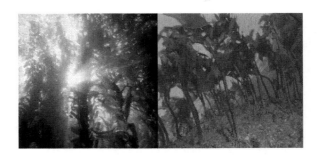

During the 19th century a French doctor named René Quinton discovered that sea water is 98% identical to blood. It makes sense that the latest and potentially most-beneficial, most well-researched, life-changing nutrient has come from the sea. Ecklonia Cava's benefits are countless and the research is staggering.

100 Times Stronger & 2400% Longer Than Green Tea!

The potency of an antioxidant is often determined by its molecular structure, which is made up of rings. Most antioxidants have **three connected rings**. Ecklonia Cava has up to **eight interconnected rings**, making its free-radical scavenging ability 10X-100X times more powerful than other antioxidants.

Up To 12 Hours Of Antioxidant Protection!

Fat-soluble ocean nutrients like Ecklonia Cava stay in the body for an extended period of time. The half-life of Ecklonia Cava is up to 12 hours, compared to 30 minutes for water-soluble, land-based polyphenols like green tea. That means that you have up to 12 full hours of antioxidant protection roaming your body and **eliminating free radicals**.

Millions On Research

Dr. Haengwoo Lee and his team spent over 32 million dollars on research, from in vitro to animal and human studies. The results are in and they are quite extraordinary. The benefits of Ecklonia Cava are many.

Research Conducted:

- Cardiovascular health including cholesterol, blood pressure, blood flow & vascular flexibility.
- Brain function related to blood flow & oxygen supply, memory, alertness, relaxation & response to stress
- Inflammation, cartilage protection, comparison to popular inflammation medications & nerve pain
- Sexual performance & comparison to popular sexual performance drugs
- Weight management & lipid metabolism

- Nerve pain
- Allergies
- Sugar spikes & pancreas support
- Sleeplessness

The Blood-Brain Barrier

Because it is fat-soluble, Ecklonia Cava also has the ability to cross the blood-brain barrier. This allows antioxidants to work in ways that traditional water-soluble antioxidants can not. Ecklonia Cava can penetrate deep into the fatty tissues of the body where much of the **acidifying toxicity hides**.

Ecklonia cava is not only superior to all land based antioxidants, it may be the king of the sea too. Also known as a sea polyphenol, Ecklonia's super powers emanate from its unique molecular structure that acts as a master switch, activating key genes, such as Nrf2, that turn on a universal network of anti-oxidant and anti-inflammatory processes to defend your body against a broad spectrum of "cellular assassins".

The result is improved brain, heart, breast, prostate, joint and overall health, with a stronger immune system and greater physical (including sexual) vitality.

You might be wondering where you can find Ecklonia Cava. The good news is that it is actually available from quite a few suppliers:

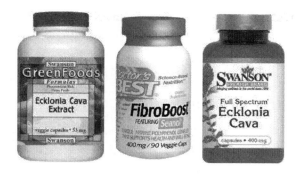

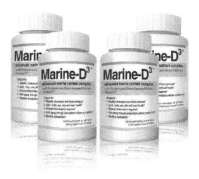

Chapter 6

Your Defensive Army of Enzymes to kill Cancer Cells

*"Life is like riding a bicycle. To keep **your balance**, you **must keep moving**."*

Albert Einstein

Now I would like you to understand a connection between low levels of ***enzymes and cancer cell growth***. Actually doctors in Europe and some doctors in the United States have used enzyme therapy with great results against cancers and have literally used enzymes to digest cancer cells.

In the early 1900's Dr. John Beard discovered that pancreatic enzymes destroy cancer cells. Making some brilliant observations, he deduced that cancer cells come from stem cells that become uncontrolled stem cells. He noticed that the fetal pancreas starts working and secreting enzymes at the 56th day of gestation. Fetuses don't digest anything till they are born. Dr. Beard wondered why the pancreas in the fetus started working so early. He noticed that the day the pancreas started producing enzymes was the day the placenta stopped growing. The enzymes stopped this rapid growth.

His theory about **enzymes and cancer** was that many placental cells remain in our body. When these misplaced placental cells get lost, they can start growing, turning cancerous if you don't have enough pancreatic enzymes. (By the way the medical community thought Dr. Beard was crazy. Now a hundred years later, medical science has confirmed the existence of these cells.)

In 1911 Dr Beard tested pancreatic enzymes for cancer prevention in mice and it worked. Unfortunately, he was blackballed by his colleagues and died in obscurity. Decades later Dr. Kelly read about his work, cured himself of cancer using pancreatic enzymes and started treating and curing many cancer patients using pancreatic enzymes. Dr. Gonzales, who has been investigating nutritional approaches to cancer and other degenerative diseases since 1981 and has been in practice in New York since 1987, went to investigate Dr. Kelly and liked what he saw so much that he also treats cancer using pancreatic enzymes.

In summary, the major reason enzyme levels become depleted in the body is that we eat mostly processed, undernourished, irradiated and cooked food full of sugars and empty carbohydrates like white flour, etc. Big increases of soy food consumption are playing a great role too. We will go much deeper into understanding how soy foods impact our health a bit later. You will be surprised to see how much soy and soybean oil and soy lecithin is sneaked into the food we buy. Unfortunately unless you carefully read the whole list of ingredients - which is usually printed in such small type that a lot of people have difficulty reading it - most of us are unaware that we are eating food products containing soy. I would strongly recommend that you carefully read the list of ingredients of each product you consider buying when doing your food shopping. It's only an investment of time the first time you do it; subsequently you will know what the healthy choices are for you the next time.

Our digestive system was designed to process **raw food**. Raw food, when it is picked **ripe and organic**, has enzymes in it that help break down that food in the upper stomach where it sits for about 30 to 45 minutes. The enzymes in the food predigest that food. Then in the lower stomach the pancreas, when healthy and functioning as it should, excretes more enzymes. Dairy products damage very much the health of the pancreas.

When we eat cooked, undernourished, irradiated and processed foods, most of the enzymes have been killed and the food does not predigest in the upper stomach. So when it reaches the lower stomach *two things happen*. The pancreas must make **extra enzymes** to try and break down the food.

And often food is only partially digested due to poor pancreas function and also to the cold drinks with ice that a lot of people consume these days while eating.

The pancreas, after decades of overworking, eventually is no longer able to produce an adequate supply of enzymes. So you develop **low levels** of all types of enzymes, and your body then *cannot* naturally kill cancer cells using enzymes.

You will be surprised but, in addition, food that is not completely digested all very often makes its way into our bloodstream. This happens especially when people have leaky gut syndrome from **candida** overgrowth. This partially digest food is treated as a toxin, and the immune system has to get rid of it. This puts an additional strain on the already overworked immune system.

Studies have found that the immune system treats the ingestion of cooked food as a toxic poison, causing a jump in white blood cells in an attempt to get rid of it as fast as possible.

"Enzymes dissolve the protein and sugar coating of the cancer cell making it vulnerable to the attack of white blood cells." This has been known since **1905 (Griffin, page 81).**

*"Fresh **Papaya** is a good **source of enzymes**. You have the papaya melons as the source of the enzyme Papain. The damasking effect of these enzymes against the pericellular layer of the malignant cell is something very concrete in the immunology of cancer. Now I prefer, rather than advising the use of papaya tablets, that the individual seeking these enzymes get them directly from the fresh papaya fruit. You have nothing to lose by eating fresh papaya melons."-* **Dr. Krebs, Jr.**

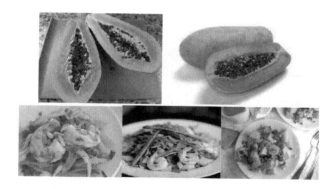

Dietary sources of all kinds of enzymes are good, and the consumption of at least 70% fresh foods vs. 30% cooked foods helps **ensure a supply of healthy enzymes** for the body (cooking at temperatures above 116°F destroys enzymes in the food). Fresh foods generally contain all the enzymes required for their own digestion, easing the burden on the digestive system. However, certain foods are more easily digested when cooked because heat breaks down starch (potatoes, for example). Cooking softens cellulose, making foods easier to chew and this, in turn, makes nutrients more available. However, **juicing** as we discussed above, also breaks down cellulose and frees the nutrients while retaining the **enzymes** that would be destroyed by cooking.

Unsprouted seeds contain enzyme inhibitors, which can be neutralized by cooking. However, soaking or sprouting the seeds also removes the enzyme inhibitors and **sprouts have a high concentration of vegetable enzymes and other nutrients**. Therefore, it is a good idea to soak your grains and beans in water for a minimum of 12 hours before eating them. Soaked grains and beans are called "pre-sprouts" and are much more digestible because the enzyme inhibitors have been deactivated. Allowing the seeds to sprout for three days allows the synthesis of new proteins, plus there is a dramatic increase in the vitamins and essential fatty acids within the sprouts.

Cooking food thoroughly kills bacteria and viruses, which is why with raw foods cleanliness becomes very important. The temperature of food and beverages also makes a difference to digestion. Warm food relaxes the stomach and aids digestion. **Cold food** and **beverages** contract the muscles of the stomach, **hindering proper digestion**.

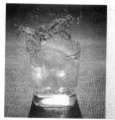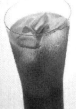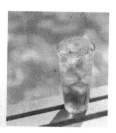

Actually it's quite dangerous for our digestive system to have cold drinks with meals. **Drink water or organic fruits and vegetable juices between meals and stop 15 min before the meal and start drinking again 40-45 min after the meal.** Beverages interfere with digestion because the **digestive liquid** and **enzymes** get carried **out** with the beverage rather than staying in the stomach. Also, drinking beverages might wash down food that has **not been properly broken** down through chewing and mixing with saliva in the mouth. This is certainly a way to create an environment to encourage colon cancer.

Lightly steaming vegetables warms and softens them while retaining most of their enzymes and nutrients.

Chapter 7

What your White Cells Want You To Know

*"So often we **dwell** on the things that **seem impossible** rather than on the things that **are possible**."*

Marian Wright Edelman

Unfortunately for the body's natural defensive mechanisms, **cancer cells** are invariably coated with and protected by **mucus and fibrin**. Our goal is to dissolve the coating that will allow our white blood cells army to perform!

Mucus is a glycoprotein (**sugar** and **protein**). **Fibrin** is a **protein** floating in the blood that allows blood to clot. This (biofilm) camouflage of mucus and fibrin prevents the white blood cells of the immune system from **recognizing the cancer cells**. Now you see the connection with why too much meat and animal protein generally in the diet is very dangerous for us. Too much animal protein in the diet as well as refined foods such as **white sugar** and **white flour** deplete pancreatic enzymes (I'll explain in more detail below), as a result helping to open the way for cancer.

Fibrin is also a contributing factor in cardiovascular disease. **Plaque** that builds up on the walls of blood vessels consists of cholesterol, cellular waste, calcium and fibrin. The plaque thickens the vessel wall, while the fibrin and **calcium** harden and cause the wall to lose critical elasticity.

For proper calcium absorption, you need to consume food sources that contain types of calcium that are easily digested, assimilated, and absorbed. It's important to know the special relationship between **magnesium** and **calcium**, as they rely on each other, and **both need** to be present for **proper absorption** as you learned above. Just for you to remember it's in a 2:1 ratio, with two parts calcium to one part of magnesium. One cup of 1-percent low-fat milk provides 305 mg of calcium and 27 mg of magnesium.
Because of the calcium-magnesium ratio in **dairy products**, our bodies **do not properly absorb** the **calcium** it contains.

A lot of us may or may not know that vegetables, legumes, whole grains, beans, lentils, and nuts contain complete protein, which is different from animal protein. Proteins can be harnessed from many plant sources. Even if you're a vegetarian, you can have alternative protein sources from plant products. The trick is, plant proteins are said to contain almost the same protein value like the ones coming from animals. The advantage is that plants are regarded as excellent sources of vitamins, minerals, fibers and antioxidants that **no animal source can match**.

Common vegetables have protein that you need, and they're complete proteins as well.

According to official sources **we need only 2.5 to 11% of our calories from protein** and common vegetables easily supply that amount. Vegetables average around 22% protein, beans 28%, and grains 13%.

Professional estimates suggest we need as little as 2.5% of our calories from protein. The U.S. government's recommendation is 5-11%, based on various factors.

The World Health Organization recommends a similar amount. And the official recommendations are padded with generous safety margins, to cover people who need more protein than average.

In general, **plant proteins** have **no cholesterol** and fat (saturated fats) as opposed to **animal sources**. That's why if you compare a person who is taking proteins from plants to someone who consumes proteins from animal sources, you can expect the latter to be more likely to develop diseases related to the **heart**, **blood pressure**, etc. and also to be more at risk of increased amounts of **fibrin** floating in the blood that can eventually cover more and more cancer cells making it impossible for white cells to recognize and kill them.

Plant proteins also have more Beta-carotene, dietary fiber, Vitamin C, Vitamin E, Folate, Iron, Magnesium and Calcium, etc. as you may have read in the charts above.

As you know, chemotherapy and radiation treatments kill cancer cells in the body as well as some **healthy cells**. We should pay particular attention during these treatments to more sensitive areas of the body like the throat, mouth area and gastro-intestinal tract. Chemotherapy also causes the immune system to overreact and excessive mucus is often the result.

Quiet often one of the side effects of chemotherapy is mucositis.

Mucositis occurs when cancer treatments break down the rapidly divided epithelial cells lining the gastro-intestinal tract, leaving the mucosal tissue open to ulceration and infection. Mucosal tissue, also known as mucosa or the mucous membrane, lines all body passages that communicate with the air, such as the respiratory and alimentary tracts, and have cells and associated glands that secrete **mucus**. The part of this lining that covers the mouth is one of the most sensitive parts of the body and is **particularly vulnerable** to chemotherapy and radiation.

The combination of mucus, excess saliva and pain can make it difficult to eat.

To reduce the production of mucus as much as possible please make sure of avoiding any consumption of mucus-producing **dairy products** like milk, cheese, yogurt of any kind, cream and ice cream. This avoidance of dairy products applies to goat dairy products as well.

Dairy products cause the body to produce mucus, especially in the gastro-intestinal tract. **In the human colon**, beta-casomorphin-7 (beta-CM-7), an exorphin derived from the **breakdown of dairy products, stimulates mucus production** from the MUC5AC gene.
This gene has been linked to **mucus hypersecretion** in the pulmonary tracts.

Cow's milk (dairy products - milk, cheese, yogurts of any kind, cream, ice cream and goat products) and fibrin (animal protein like beef, pork etc.) are notoriously the most **cancer-coating foods** we can consume.

Casein, the protein component in milk, is a very thick and coarse substance and is used to make one of the strongest glues known to man. There is **300%** more casein in cows' milk than in human milk.

The **casein** in cows' milk can **clog** and **irritate** the body's **entire respiratory system**. Dairy products are implicated in almost all respiratory problems. Hay fever, asthma, bronchitis, sinusitis, colds, runny noses and ear infections can all be caused by the consumption of dairy products. Dairy products are also the leading cause of allergies.

"There is compelling evidence, now published in top scientific journals and some of which is decades old, showing that cows' milk is associated, possibly even causally, with a wide variety of serious human ailments including various cancers, cardiovascular diseases, diabetes and an array of allergy-related diseases. And, this food contains no nutrients that cannot be better obtained from other far more nutritious and tasty foods." Dr. Colin Campbell

"Inclusion of milk will only reduce your diet's nutritional value and safety. Most of the people on the planet live very healthfully without cow's milk. You can too." Robert M. Kradjian M.D

"I no longer recommend dairy products...there was a time when cow's milk was considered very desirable. But research along with clinical experience has forced doctors

and nutritionists to rethink this recommendation" Dr. Benjamin Spock

*According to Dr. Julian Whitaker in his 'Health & Healing' newsletter in an article entitled 'Tomorrow's Medicine Today' (October 1998 Vol. 8, No. 10) the notion that milk is healthy for you is "udder" nonsense. While eating fruits, vegetables and whole grains has been documented to lower the risk of heart attack, high blood pressure and cancer, the widely touted health benefits of dairy products are questionable at best. In fact, **dairy products** are clearly linked as a **cause** of **osteoporosis, heart disease, obesity, cancer, allergies and diabetes**. He argues that dairy products are anything but "health" foods.*

If you are a big fan of dairy products and love drinking milk by itself or with cereals, I recommend you replace dairy products with very delicious non-dairy alternatives such as **Almond Milk, Brown Rice Milk, Hazelnut Milk, Quinoa Milk, Oat Milk and others made of cereals and nuts. Be careful to avoid any form of Soy Milk.**

Chapter 8

Food Containing Soy

*"Anyone who stops learning is old, whether at twenty or eighty. Anyone who keeps learning stays young. **The greatest thing in life is to keep your mind young."***

Henry Ford

Soybeans contain natural toxins that inhibit protein digestion in the body and should be completely avoided in your foods going forward. Only a few decades ago, unfermented soybean foods were considered unfit to eat - even in Asia. These days, people all over the world have been fooled into thinking that unfermented soy foods like soymilk and soy protein are somehow "health foods". If they only knew the real truth!

The soybean did not serve as a food until the discovery of fermentation techniques, sometime during the Chou Dynasty. The first soy foods were fermented products like tempeh, natto, miso and soy sauce.

At a later date, possibly in the 2nd century BC, Chinese scientists discovered that a puree of cooked soybeans could be precipitated with calcium sulphate or magnesium sulphate to make a smooth, pale curd - tofu or bean curd. The use of fermented and precipitated soy products soon spread to other parts of the Orient, notably Japan and Indonesia.

Growth-depressant compounds are deactivated during the process of fermentation, so once the Chinese discovered how to ferment the soybean, they began to incorporate soy foods into their diets.

The Chinese NEVER ate large amounts of unfermented soy foods or soymilk.

The Chinese did not eat unfermented soybeans as they did other legumes such as lentils because the soybean contains large quantities of natural toxins or "anti nutrients". First among them are potent enzyme inhibitors that **block the action of trypsin and other enzymes vital for protein digestion.**

These inhibitors are large, tightly folded proteins that are not completely deactivated during ordinary cooking. They can produce serious gastric distress, reduced protein digestion and chronic deficiencies in amino acid uptake. In test animals, diets high in trypsin inhibitors cause enlargement and pathological conditions of the pancreas, including cancer.

Soybeans also contain **haemagglutinin**, a clot-promoting substance that **causes red blood cells to clump together**. Trypsin inhibitors and haemagglutinin are growth inhibitors. Weaned rats fed soy containing these antinutrients fail to grow normally.

Soy also contains **goitrogens** - substances that depress **thyroid function**.

Although soy has been known to suppress thyroid function for over 60 years, and although scientists have identified the goitrogenic component of soy as the so-called "beneficial isoflavones", the industry insists that soy depresses thyroid function only in the absence of iodine.

The University of Alabama at Birmingham reports a case in which consumption of a soy protein dietary supplement decreased the absorption of thyroxin. The patient had undergone thyroid surgery and needed to take thyroid hormone. Higher oral doses of thyroid hormone were needed when she consumed soy - she presumably used iodized salt so iodine intake did not prevent the goitrogenic effects of soy.

A very large percentage of soy is genetically modified and it also has one of the highest percentages of **contamination by pesticides** of any of our foods.

Soybeans are high in phytic acid, present in the bran or hulls of all seeds. Phytic acid is a substance that can block the uptake of essential minerals - **calcium, magnesium, copper, iron and especially zinc - in the intestinal tract.**
The soybean has one of the highest phytate levels of any grain or legume that has been studied, and the phytates in soy are highly resistant to normal phytate-reducing techniques such as long, slow cooking. Only a long period of fermentation will significantly reduce the phytate content of soybeans.

Soy Protein Isolate (SPI) is an Industrially Produced Food - Far from Natural or Healthy!

SPI is not something you can make in your own kitchen. Production takes place in industrial factories where slurry of soy beans is first mixed with an alkaline solution to remove fibre, then precipitated and separated using an acid wash and, finally, neutralized in an alkaline solution.

Acid washing in aluminium tanks leaches high levels of aluminium into the final product. The resultant curds are spray-dried at high temperatures to produce a high-protein powder. A final indignity to the original soybean is high-temperature; high-pressure extrusion processing of soy protein isolates to produce textured vegetable protein.

In feeding experiments, the use of SPI increased requirements for vitamins E, K, D and B12 and created **deficiency symptoms** of calcium, magnesium, manganese, molybdenum, copper, iron and zinc. Phytic acid remaining in these soy products greatly inhibits zinc and iron absorption; test animals fed SPI develop enlarged organs, particularly the **pancreas and thyroid gland**, and increased deposition of fatty acids in the liver.

Yet soy protein isolate and textured vegetable protein (TVP) are used extensively in school lunch programs, commercial baked goods, **diet beverages** and **fast food** products. They are heavily promoted in third world countries and form the basis of many food give-away programs.

Soy has the potential to disrupt the **digestive, immune and endocrine systems** of the human body and its role in rising rates of infertility, hypothyroidism and some types of **cancer including thyroid** and **pancreatic cancers**.

Soy is also highly **allergenic**. Most experts now place soy protein among the top eight allergens of all foods, and some rate it in the top six or even top four. Allergic reactions to soy are increasingly common, ranging from mild to life threatening, and some fatalities have been reported.

Did you know an infant fed soy formula is getting the hormonal equivalent of five birth control pills per day?

Even after rigorous chemical processing, soy contains substances that can possibly cause breast cancer, serious nutritional deficiencies, and even accelerated brain aging!

Unlike other legumes, soybeans aren't safe to eat when picked fresh. **They're actually toxic**. And in laboratory tests in animals, soybeans have been shown to cause everything from **cancer** to **birth defects**.

In order to remove the harmful toxins mentioned above, manufacturers must use harsh chemical processing. The beans are subject to acid baths and extreme heat, then they're spray dried to produce a high-protein powder. Next, to improve the taste of the soy powder, artificial flavourings such as MSG, preservatives, sweeteners, emulsifiers and synthetic nutrients are added.

Carcinogens, called nitrites, are also added to soy products during the spray drying process. These harmful chemicals are found in hot dogs and other fast foods... and they've been known since the dark ages to cause cancer. Plus, after all that...

Despite nearly 1/2 billion dollars in funding, nobody's figured out how to remove all the toxins from soybeans

That's right. There's not enough money in the world that can make soybeans as safe to eat as black beans.

The problem is, manufacturers can't get rid of all of the soybean's natural toxins. One especially dangerous toxin, called a trypsin inhibitor, can interfere with digestion and could theoretically cause cancer in humans.

In feeding experiments, a soy-based diet requires supplementation with vitamins E, K, D, B'2, and creates significant DEFICIENCIES in copper, iron, zinc, magnesium, and calcium. This revelation is especially important for postmenopausal woman. By eating quantities of soy, you could be putting yourself at risk for serious nutritional deficiencies and osteoporosis. But that's not the only concern for women eating soy...

Researchers have linked soy to an early form of breast cancer

You may have heard that eating soy can protect you from developing breast cancer. There's research to say that's so! But, to quote a famous commentator: "Here's the rest of the story!"

In one significant study completed in 1996, researchers found that women who ate soy protein had an increased incidence of epithelial hyperplasia, an early form of malignancy. A year later, a chemical found in soy was shown to **encourage breast cells to metastasize**.

You can get as much "estrogen" eating soy protein as taking the birth control pill

You may have heard that soy contains beneficial substances called isoflavones.

They're thought to improve symptoms associated with menopause. But isoflavones can also wreak havoc on your hormonal system.

Here's how...

One hundred grams of soy protein daily, the amount recommended by a national soy organization, provides the estrogenic equivalent of taking the **birth control pill**.

In 1991, Japanese researchers found that as little as two teaspoons of soy protein a day caused goiter and hyperthyroidism in some patients. Isoflavones were believed to be the culprit.

Isoflavones are also thought to cause all sorts of problems in infants. In fact, an infant who is fed soy formula is getting the estrogenic equivalent of five birth control pills a day. Some experts believe this excess estrogen can lead to thyroid problems, learning disabilities, and even premature sexual development.

That's a disturbing possibility, considering that nearly 1/2 of all bottle fed babies in the U.S. receive soy formula.

Recent research ties two or more servings a week of tofu with "accelerated brain aging"

One of the most shocking discoveries about soy came to light at the Third International Soy Symposium in 1999. On the last day of the symposium, one researcher presented his three-decade long study of Japanese-Americans living in Hawaii.

It showed a significant statistical relationship between eating two or more servings of tofu a week and "accelerated brain aging."

Individuals who ate this amount of tofu in midlife had lower cognitive function later in life and a greater incidence of Alzheimer's disease and dementia. Again, researchers believed isoflavones were the offenders.

Many of these findings were confirmed by Dr. Daniel Dorge of the Division of Biochemical Toxicology at the National Center for Toxicological Research, who is one of the nation's top soy researchers and Daniel Sheehan. (Ref. Also "True Health" Carotec, Inc. newsletter, Tom Valentine.)

I would very much recommend you to look at the ingredients when buying your foods, as you are going to be very surprised about the amount of food these days **containing SOY!**

At the same time that we should be avoiding Soy, there exists a wide variety of very healthy beans and peas available for us to enjoy while at the same time providing good levels of nourishment for our bodies:

Best Alkalizing Beans and Peas with Mineral and Vitamin content

Beans/Peas	Protein/Fiber	Minerals	Vitamins
Adzuki Beans	100 grams of Adzuki Beans, boiled without salt contain 7.52 grams protein, 128 calories and 7.3 grams dietary fiber.	Potassium - 532 mg Phosphorus - 168 mg Calcium - 28 mg Magnesium - 52 mg Iron - 2 mg Sodium - 8 mg Selenium - 1.2 mcg Zinc - 1.77 mg Manganese - 0.573 mg Copper - 0.298 mg Also contains a	Vitamin B1 (thiamine) - 0.115 mg Vitamin B2 (riboflavin) - 0.064 mg Niacin - 0.717 mg Folate - 121 mcg Pantothenic Acid - 0.430 mg Vitamin B6 - 0.096 mg Vitamin A - 6 IU Contains some other vitamins in small amounts.

		small amount of other minerals.	
Black Beans	100 grams of Black Beans, boiled without salt, contain 8.86 grams protein, 132 calories and 8.7 grams of dietary fiber.	Potassium - 355 mg Phosphorus - 140 mg Calcium - 27 mg Magnesium - 70 mg Iron - 2.1 mg Sodium - 1 mg Manganese - 0.444 mg Zinc - 1.12 mg Copper - 0.209 mg Selenium - 1.2 mcg Also contains trace amounts of other minerals.	Vitamin B1 (thiamine) - 0.244 mg Vitamin B2 (riboflavin) - 0.059 mg Niacin - 0.505 mg Pantothenic Acid - 0.242 mg Vitamin B6 - 0.069 mg Folate - 149 mcg Vitamin A - 6 IU Contains some other vitamins in small amounts.
Black Eye or Cow Peas	100 grams of cooked, Black Eye Peas contain 7.73 grams protein, 116 calories and 6.5 grams dietary fiber.	Potassium - 278 mg Phosphorus - 156 mg Calcium - 24 mg Magnesium - 53 mg Iron - 2.51 mg Sodium - 4 mg Manganese - 0.475 mg Zinc - 1.29 mg Copper - 0.268 mg Selenium - 2.5 mcg Also contains trace amounts of other minerals.	Vitamin B1 (thiamine) - 0.202 mg Vitamin B2 (riboflavin) - 0.055 mg Niacin - 0.495 mg Pantothenic Acid - 0.411 mg Vitamin B6 - 0.1 mg Folate - 208 mcg Vitamin A - 15 IU Vitamin E - 0.28 mg Vitamin K - 1.7 mcg Contains some other vitamins in small amounts.
Broad or Fava Beans	100 grams of Broad Beans contain 7.6 grams of protein, 110 calories and 5.4 grams of dietary fiber.	Potassium - 268 mg Phosphorus - 125 mg Calcium - 36 mg Magnesium - 43 mg Iron - 1.5 mg Sodium - 5 mg Manganese - 0.421 mg Zinc - 1.01 mg Copper - 0.259 mg Selenium - 2.6 mcg	Vitamin C - 0.3 mg Vitamin B1 (thiamine) - 0.097 mg Vitamin B2 (riboflavin) - 0.089 mg Niacin - 0.711 mg Pantothenic Acid - 0.157 mg Vitamin B6 - 0.072 mg Folate - 104 mcg Vitamin A - 15 IU Vitamin E - 0.02 mg

		Also contains trace amounts of other minerals.	Vitamin K - 2.9 mcg Contains some other vitamins in small amounts.
Edamame	100 grams of frozen, unprepared Edamame contain 10.25 grams protein, 110 calories and 4.8 grams dietary fiber.	Potassium - 482 mg Phosphorus - 161 mg Calcium - 60 mg Magnesium - 61 mg Iron - 2.11 mg Sodium - 6 mg Manganese - 1.01 mg Zinc - 1.32 mg Copper - 0.324 mg Also contains trace amounts of other minerals.	Vitamin C - 9.7 mg Vitamin B1 (thiamine) - 0.15 mg Vitamin B2 (riboflavin) - 0.265 mg Niacin - 0.925 mg Pantothenic Acid - 0.535 mg Vitamin B6 - 0.135 mg Folate - 303 mcg Vitamin E - 0.72 mg Vitamin K - 31.4 mcg Contains some other vitamins in small amounts.
Chick Peas/Garbanzo Beans	100 grams of Garbanzo Beans, boiled without salt contain 8.86 grams protein, 164 calories and 7.6 grams of fiber.	Potassium - 291 mg Phosphorus - 168 mg Calcium - 49 mg Magnesium - 48 mg Iron - 2.89 mg Sodium - 7 mg Manganese - 1.03 mg Zinc - 1.53 mg Copper - 0.352 mg Selenium - 3.7 mcg Also contains trace amounts of other minerals.	Vitamin C - 1.3 mg Vitamin B1 (thiamine) - 0.116 mg Vitamin B2 (riboflavin) - 0.063 mg Niacin - 0.526 mg Pantothenic Acid - 0.286 mg Vitamin B6 - 0.139 mg Folate - 172 mcg Vitamin A - 27 IU Vitamin E - 0.35 mg Vitamin K - 4 mcg Contains some other vitamins in small amounts.
Kidney or Red Beans	100 grams of Kidney Beans, boiled without salt, contain 8.67 grams of protein, 127 calories and 7.3 grams dietary fiber.	Potassium - 403 mg Phosphorus - 142 mg Calcium - 28 mg Magnesium - 45 mg Iron - 2.94 mg Sodium - 2 mg Manganese - 0.477 mg Zinc - 1.07 mg	Vitamin C - 1.2 mg Vitamin B1 (thiamine) - 0.216 mg Vitamin B2 (riboflavin) - 0.058 mg Niacin - 0.578 mg Pantothenic Acid - 0.22 mg Vitamin B6 - 0.12 mg

		Copper - 0.242 mg Selenium - 1.2 mcg Also contains trace amounts of other minerals.	Folate - 130 mcg Vitamin E - 0.03 mg Vitamin K - 8.4 mcg Contains some other vitamins in small amounts.
Lima Beans	100 grams of Lima Beans, boiled without salt contain 7.80 grams of protein, 115 calories and 7.0 grams of dietary fiber.	Potassium - 508 mg Phosphorus - 111 mg Calcium - 17 mg Magnesium - 43 mg Iron - 2.39 mg Sodium - 2 mg Manganese - 0.516 mg Zinc - 0.95 mg Copper - 0.235 mg Selenium - 4.5 mcg Also contains trace amounts of other minerals.	Vitamin B1 (thiamine) - 0.161 mg Vitamin B2 (riboflavin) - 0.055 mg Niacin - 0.421 mg Pantothenic Acid - 0.422 mg Vitamin B6 - 0.161 mg Folate - 83 mcg Vitamin E - 0.18 mg Vitamin K - 2 mcg Contains some other vitamins in small amounts.
Mung Beans	100 grams of Mung Beans, boiled without salt, have 7.02 grams of protein, 105 calories and 7.6 grams of dietary fiber.	Potassium - 266 mg Phosphorus - 99 mg Calcium - 27 mg Magnesium - 48 mg Iron - 1.4 mg Sodium - 2 mg Manganese - 0.298 mg Zinc - 0.84 mg Copper - 0.156 mg Selenium - 2.5 mcg Also contains trace amounts of other minerals.	Vitamin B1 (thiamine) - 0.164 mg Vitamin B2 (riboflavin) - 0.061 mg Niacin - 0.577 mg Pantothenic Acid - 0.41 mg Vitamin B6 - 0.067 mg Folate - 159 mcg Vitamin A - 24 IU Vitamin E - 0.15 mg Vitamin K - 2.7 mcg Contains some other vitamins in small amounts.
Navy Beans	100 grams Navy Beans, boiled without salt contain 8.23 grams proteins, 140 calories and 10.5 grams of dietary fiber.	Potassium - 389 mg Phosphorus - 144 mg Calcium - 69 mg Magnesium - 53 mg Iron - 2.36 mg Manganese - 0.527 mg Zinc - 1.03 mg	Vitamin C - 0.9 mg Vitamin B1 (thiamine) - 0.237 mg Vitamin B2 (riboflavin) - 0.066 mg Niacin - 0.649 mg Pantothenic Acid - 0.266 mg Vitamin B6 - 0.138

		Copper - 0.21 mg Selenium - 2.9 mcg Also contains trace amounts of other minerals.	mg Folate - 140 mcg Vitamin E - 0.01 mg Vitamin K - 0.6 mcg Contains some other vitamins in small amounts.
Pigeon Peas	100 grams of Pigeon Peas boiled without salt contain 6.76 grams proteins, 121 calories and 6.7 grams of dietary fiber.	Potassium -384 mg Phosphorus - 119 mg Calcium - 43 mg Magnesium - 46 mg Iron - 1.11 mg Sodium - 5 mg Manganese - 0.501 mg Zinc - 0.9 mg Copper - 0.269 mg Selenium - 2.9 mcg Also contains trace amounts of other minerals.	Vitamin B1 (thiamine) - 0.146 mg Vitamin B2 (riboflavin) - 0.059 mg Niacin - 0.781 mg Pantothenic Acid - 0.319 mg Vitamin B6 - 0.05 mg Folate - 111 mcg Vitamin A - 3 IU Contains some other vitamins in small amounts.
Pinto Beans	100 grams of Pinto Beans, boiled without salt, contain 9.01 grams of protein, 143 calories and 9 grams fiber.	Potassium - 436 mg Phosphorus - 147 mg Calcium - 46 mg Magnesium - 50 mg Iron - 2.09 mg Sodium - 1 mg Manganese - 0.453 mg Zinc - 0.98 mg Copper - 0.219 mg Selenium - 6.2 mcg Also contains trace amounts of other minerals.	Vitamin C - 0.8 mg Vitamin B1 (thiamine) - 0.193 mg Vitamin B2 (riboflavin) - 0.062 mg Niacin - 0.318 mg Pantothenic Acid - 0.21 mg Vitamin B6 - 0.229 mg Folate - 172 mcg Vitamin E - 0.94 mg Vitamin K - 3.5 mcg Contains some other vitamins in small amounts.
Split Peas	100 grams of Split Peas, boiled, without salt contain 8.34 grams protein, 118 calories and 8.3 grams dietary fiber.	Potassium - 362 mg Phosphorus - 99 mg Calcium - 14 mg Magnesium - 36 mg Iron - 1.29 mg Sodium - 2 mg Manganese -	Vitamin C - 0.4 mg Vitamin B1 (thiamine) - 0.19 mg Vitamin B2 (riboflavin) - 0.056 mg Niacin - 0.89 mg Pantothenic Acid - 0.595 mg

		0.396 mg Zinc - 1 mg Copper - 0.181 mg Selenium - 0.6 mcg Also contains trace amounts of other minerals.	Vitamin B6 - 0.048 mg Folate - 65 mcg Vitamin A - 7 IU Vitamin E - 0.03 mg Vitamin K - 5 mcg Contains some other vitamins in small amounts.
White Beans	100 grams White Beans, boiled without salt, contain 8.97 grams protein, 142 calories and 10.4 grams dietary fiber.	Potassium - 463 mg Phosphorus - 169 mg Calcium - 73 mg Magnesium - 68 mg Iron - 2.84 mg Manganese - 0.51 mg Zinc - 1.09 mg Copper - 0.149 mg Selenium - 1.3 mcg Also contains trace amounts of other minerals.	Vitamin B1 (thiamine) - 0.236 mg Vitamin B2 (riboflavin) - 0.059 mg Niacin - 0.272 mg Pantothenic Acid - 0.251 mg Vitamin B6 - 0.127 mg Folate - 137 mcg Contains some other vitamins in small amounts.
Winged Beans	100 grams Winged Beans, boiled without salt, contain 10.62 grams of protein and 147 calories.	Potassium - 280 mg Phosphorus - 153 mg Calcium - 142 mg Magnesium - 54 mg Iron - 4.33 mg Sodium - 13 mg Manganese - 1.199 mg Zinc - 1.44 mg Copper - 0.773 mg Selenium - 2.9 mcg Also contains trace amounts of other minerals.	Vitamin B1 (thiamine) - 0.295 mg Vitamin B2 (riboflavin) - 0.129 mg Niacin - 0.83 mg Pantothenic Acid - 0.156 mg Vitamin B6 - 0.047 mg Folate - 10 mcg Contains some other vitamins in small amounts.

Chapter 9

Our Body's Powerhouse

*"The world as we have created it is **a process** of our* **thinking. It cannot be changed without changing our thinking."**

Albert Einstein

To help our bodies with **growing only new, healthy cells** and to **strengthen only existing healthy cells**, we need to understand the vital part played by **Mitochondria**.

Mitochondria, which are tiny structures inside our body's cells, **are the powerhouse of our cells.**

Mitochondria are essentially the biological engines that convert **carbohydrates**, **proteins** and **fats** into the energy required and consumed by the entire body. **Efficient mitochondria** provide the **energy** for our **cells** and keep our cells **healthy**. Healthy cells are the **key** to a whole range of benefits for our brain and body, including increased energy levels.

"The main function of the mitochondrion is the production

of energy, in the form of adenosine triphosphate (ATP). The cell uses this energy to perform the specific work necessary for cell survival and function.

*The raw materials used to generate ATP are the **foods** that we eat, or tissues within the body that are broken down in a process called catabolism. The breaking down of food into simpler molecules such as **carbohydrates, fats**, and **protein** is called **metabolism**. These molecules are then transferred into the **mitochondria**, where further processing occurs. The reactions within the mitochondria produce specific molecules that can have their electrical charges separated within the inner mitochondrial membrane. These charged molecules are processed within the five electron transport chain complexes to finally combine with oxygen to make ATP. The process of the charged substances combining with oxygen is called **oxidation**, while the chemical reaction making ATP is called phosphorylation. The overall process is called oxidative phosphorylation. The product produced by this process is ATP.*

*Cell death can occur either by injury due to **toxic exposure**, by mechanical damage, or by an orderly process called **programmed cell death** or **apoptosis**. Programmed cell death occurs during development as the organism is pruning away unwanted, excess cells. It also occurs during infections with viruses**, cancer therapy**, or in the **immune response to illness**. The process of programmed cell death is another function of **mitochondria**.*

*Normally, ATP production is coupled to oxygen consumption. During abnormal states such as fever, **cancer**, or **stroke**, or when dysfunction occurs within the* *mitochondria, more oxygen is consumed or **required** than is actually used to make ATP. The mitochondria become partially "uncoupled" and produce **highly reactive oxygen species called free radicals.** When the production of free radicals overwhelms the mitochondria's ability to **"detoxify"** them, the excess free radicals damage mitochondrial function by changing the **mitochondrial DNA**, proteins, and membranes. As this process continues, it can induce the cell to undergo **apoptosis**. Abnormal cell death due to mitochondrial dysfunction can interfere with organ function.*

***Mitochondria** are involved in **building, breaking down,** and **recycling products** needed for **proper cell functioning**. For example, some of the building blocks of DNA and RNA occur within the mitochondria. Mitochondria are also involved in making parts of blood and hormones such as **estrogen** and **testosterone**. They are required for **cholesterol metabolism, neurotransmitter metabolism, and detoxification** of ammonia in the urea cycle. **Thus, if mitochondria do not function properly, not only energy production but also cell-specific products needed for normal cell functioning will be affected."** By Russell P. Saneto, D.O., Ph.D., Children's Hospital and Regional Medical Center/University of Washington School of Medicine, Seattle, WA.*

Mitochondria were first proposed to be relevant to cancer by Nobel prize-winner Dr Otto Warburg who reported that cancer cells exhibited "aerobic-glycolysis". Although this was originally interpreted as indicating that the function of mitochondria was defective, we now understand that cancer cells are in an altered metabolic state.

From the information you have read above, you can appreciate the **crucial importance** of the **quality of the food** we are providing to our bodies to achieve and sustain good health, the overall quality of our life and the quality of our brain power and energy levels we desire to experience every day of our life. By giving **good quality nutritional material** for our **cells to work with** (food that we consume every day) we give our cells the opportunity to do their job properly. You only have to provide the best raw material and they will do an excellent job for you! Our body is an intelligent, complex factory, requiring very **high quality materials** in order to continue to produce very **high quality results in the form of perfect, uncompromised replacement cells**!

Mitochondria are probably the most important structures found in cells. They make up as much as 60% of the volume of muscle cells and 40% of the volume of **heart cells**. They are involved in almost every energy intensive process in the cell and many diseases that deal with energy balances (**diabetes, sarcopenia, cancer, multiple sclerosis**) can be traced back to defects in a cell's mitochondria. In fact, mitochondria are so important to the survival of the cell that they even contain their own DNA so they don't have to depend on the nucleus to repair or replace themselves.

As a great example of the power of Mitochondria, here is the extraordinary and true story about Professor of Medicine Dr. Terry Wahls MD after she was diagnosed with Multiple Sclerosis.

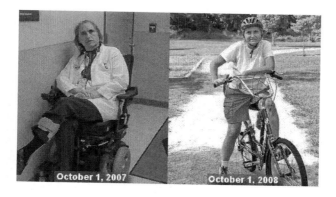

As you will read, Dr. Terry Wahls decided to pay attention to the important role **mitochondria plays in our overall health** and actually cured herself by changing her nutrition much the same way that you will be changing yours. Her main shift was a change in her daily diet. She included lots of green organic vegetables (**alkalizing**) that you saw in the book chart above, grass-fed meat (you can have fish, preferably local catch or any wild fish available at your local supermarket, ideally not more than a couple of times a week). She also avoided foods that contain too much acidity.

Here is Dr. Terry Wahl's story in her own words:
"...I am a clinical professor of medicine at the University of Iowa Carver College of Medicine in Iowa City, Iowa, U.S.A., where I teach internal medicine residents in their primary care clinics. I also do clinical research and have published over 60 peer-reviewed scientific abstracts, posters and papers.

In addition to being a doctor, I am also a patient with a chronic, progressive disease. I was diagnosed with relapsing remitting multiple sclerosis in 2000, just as I began working for the University. By 2003 I had transitioned to secondary progressive multiple sclerosis. I underwent chemotherapy in an attempt to slow the disease and began using a tilt-recline wheelchair because of weakness in my back muscles. It was clear: eventually I would become bedridden by my disease. I wanted to forestall that fate as long as possible.

Because of my academic medical training, I know that research in animal models of disease is often 20 or 30 years ahead of clinical practice. Hoping to find something to arrest my descent into becoming bedridden, I used PubMed.gov to begin searching the scientific articles about the latest multiple sclerosis research. Night after night, I relearned biochemistry, cellular physiology, and neuroimmunology to understand the articles. Unfortunately, most of the studies were testing drugs that were years away from FDA approval. Then it occurred to me to search for vitamins and supplements that helped any kind of progressive brain disorder. Slowly I created a list of nutrients important to brain health and began taking them as supplements. The steepness of my decline slowed, for which I was grateful, but I still was declining.

In the fall of 2007, I had an important epiphany. What if I redesigned my diet so that I was getting those important brain nutrients not from supplements but from the foods I ate? It took more time to create this new diet, intensive directed nutrition, which I designed to provide optimal nutrition for my brain. At that time, I also learned about neuromuscular electrical stimulation and convinced my physical therapist to give me a test session. It hurt, a lot, but I also felt euphoric when it was finished, likely because of the endorphins my body released in response to the electrical stimulation. In December 2007, I began my intensive directed nutrition along with a program of progressive exercise, electrical stimulation, and daily meditation. The results stunned my physician, my family and me: within a year, I was able to walk through the hospital without a cane and even complete an 18-mile bicycle tour.

In 2007 I was losing my phone and keys and was afraid my chief of staff would soon be calling me to his office to tell me that it was time to revoke my clinical privileges. I expected to become ever more dependent because of my illness. Instead, within a year of starting my regimen I regained the ability to commute to work on my bicycle, do my rounds on foot without canes or wheelchairs, conduct clinical trials and write grants, all by making changes to the foods I ate and keeping up with exercise and stress management…"

Thanks to Dr. Terry Wahls's own research, knowledge and decision to fight and win the disease and get healthy, she was able in a period of **one year** to exchange a **wheel chair** for a **bicycle** and even enjoy **horse riding**.

Dr Wahls body was given the right nutritional resources to recover her health. Hopefully You are also clearly motivated to make the decision to make changes to your diet and to say a permanent "NO" to a few food types you probably liked to eat very much in your past and replace them with the far more healthy options that you have now learned that exist for all of us and that are available to you in reference for in the earlier tables I shared with you.

God gave each of us such a wonderful gift – the gift of choice…so please ask yourself what is your choice now? Take a few minutes, sit very quietly and try to look inside your beautiful soul and decide what your **choice is now for the health of your body which sustains your life**?

You have the power and knowledge needed to live a longer and healthier life. You understand now that you **can** protect yourself, fight and beat cancer disease because you know how to create an alkaline body environment that prevents cancer cells from surviving and being active. So it is time to make that choice and use your mind and will power to create a "super climate" in your body for your healthy cells to have as much cancer neutralizing power as you can give them. **You have no idea how much your cells will pay you in return.** Just provide them with the necessary environment to function at their best. Our body was designed by a very intelligent source and, like most complex machines, it's ability to operate perfectly is very sensitive to the type of "fuel" we give it; depending on **what** and **how much** you decide to help it, it can **destroy** itself or it can **heal** itself!

We are coming now to the book chart about fruits and before we do, I would like to share with you a few ideas you can use in your kitchen to provide yourself and may be your loved ones with some delicious and healthy meals that many of you will find delicious.

Shrimp and Mango Salad

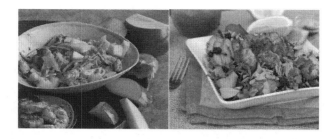

This salad is delicious served immediately at room temperature. It's even better after being chilled for an hour to combine the flavors.

Ingredients:

1 pound **grilled shrimp**, chopped
3 large mangoes, peeled and cut into chunks
1/2 small red onion, thinly sliced
3 tablespoons chopped cilantro
1/2 jalapeño pepper, seeded and chopped (optional)
Juice of 2 large limes
Sea salt to taste

Preparation:

1 Place all the ingredients but the salt in a large bowl. Stir to combine.
2 Season with the sea salt and serve.

Organic Chicken, Avocado and Mango Salad

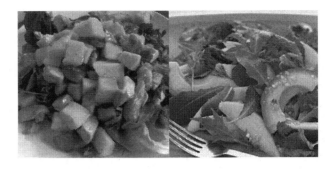

Ingredients:

For 2 servings:

1 cup shredded, cooked organic chicken
   1 tablespoon water
   1 tablespoon and 1 teaspoon lime juice
   2 tablespoons chili garlic sauce
1/2 medium mangos - peeled, seeded and diced
   1/2 avocados - peeled, pitted and diced
   1/4 (10 ounce) package spring lettuce mix
1-teaspoon brown sugar or honey

Directions:

In a saucepan over medium-high heat, stir together the brown sugar or honey and water. Bring to a boil, then pour into a medium bowl. Stir in the garlic chili sauce and lime juice. Set the dressing aside.

In a large bowl, toss together organic chicken, mangos and avocados. Arrange the spring salad mix on serving plates, then top with a few spoonfuls of the chicken mixture. Pour dressing over the top.

Avocado and Papaya Salad with Lime Dressing

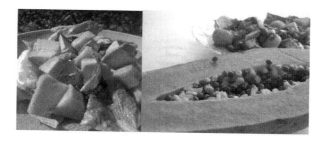

INGREDIENTS :

2 papayas
2 avocados
2 limes, juiced
1 tablespoon honey
1/4 teaspoon sea salt
1/4 teaspoon freshly cracked black pepper
4 cups mixed baby lettuce greens

PREPARATIONS

1. Combine the lime juice, honey, sea salt and pepper; blend until smooth.

2. Peel the papayas and cut them in half. Using a spoon, remove the seeds; discard seeds.

3. Slice the papaya halves into thin wedges. Cut the avocados in half and remove the pits. Slice the flesh into thin strips.

4. Arrange the fruit slices on salad plates, alternating

between papaya and avocado.

5. Combine the greens and dressing in a bowl and toss well to coat.

6. Mound a portion of the greens in the center of each plate. Drizzle with a few drops of dressing.

You probably are curious and interested in the full list of fruits that are healthy to eat on their own or for making salads and other dishes with and just as importantly, just to make delicious, healthy juices from... Here they are for you! All fruits shown below should be consumed ripe and preferably grown organically.

Best Alkalizing Fruits with Mineral and Vitamin content

Fruits	Amount	Minerals Contained	Vitamins Contained
Apple	One medium apple with skin contains 0.47 grams of protein, 95 calories, and 4.4 grams of dietary fiber.	Potassium - 195 mg Calcium - 11 mg Phosphorus - 20 mg Magnesium - 9 mg Manganese - 0.064 mg Iron - 0.22 mg Sodium - 2 mg Copper - 0.049 mg Zinc - 0.07 mg Also contains a trace amount of other minerals.	Vitamin A - 98 IU Vitamin B1 (thiamine) - 0.031 mg Vitamin B2 (riboflavin) - 0.047 mg Niacin - 0.166 mg Folate - 5 mcg Pantothenic Acid - 0.111 mg Vitamin B6 - 0.075 mg Vitamin C - 8.4 mg Vitamin E - 0.33 mg Vitamin K - 4 mcg Contains some other vitamins in small amounts.

Avocado	One medium avocado contains 4.02 grams of protein, 322 calories and 13.5 grams of fiber.	Potassium - 975 mg Phosphorus - 105 mg Magnesium - 58 mg Calcium - 24 mg Sodium - 14 mg Iron - 1.11 mg Selenium 0.8 mcg Manganese - 0.285 mg Copper - 0.382 mg Zinc - 1.29 mg Also contains small amounts of other minerals.	Vitamin A - 293 IU Vitamin C - 20.1 mg Vitamin B1 (thiamine) - 0.135 mg Vitamin B2 (riboflavin) - 0.261 mg Niacin - 3.493 mg Folate - 163 mcg Pantothenic Acid - 2.792 mg Vitamin B6 - .517 mg Vitamin E - 4.16 mg Vitamin K - 42.2 mcg Contains some other vitamins in small amounts.
Banana	One medium banana contains 1.29 grams of protein, 105 calories and 3.1 grams of dietary fiber.	Potassium - 422 mg Phosphorus - 26 mg Magnesium - 32 mg Calcium - 6 mg Sodium - 1 mg Iron - 0.31 mg Selenium 1.2 mcg Manganese - 0.319 mg Copper - 0.092 mg Zinc - 0.18 mg Also contains small amounts of other minerals.	Vitamin A - 76 IU Vitamin B1 (thiamine) - 0.037 mg Vitamin B2 (riboflavin) - 0.086 mg Niacin - 0.785 mg Folate - 24 mcg Pantothenic Acid - 0.394 mg Vitamin B6 - 0.433 mg Vitamin C - 10.3 mg Vitamin E - 0.12 mg Vitamin K - 0.6 mcg Contains some other vitamins in small amounts.
Blackberries	One cup of blackberries contains 2 grams of protein, 62 calories and 7.6 grams of dietary fiber.	Potassium - 233 mg Phosphorus - 32 mg Magnesium - 29 mg Calcium - 42 mg Sodium - 1 mg Iron - 0.89 mg Selenium 0.6 mcg Manganese - 0.93 mg Copper - 0.238	Vitamin A - 308 IU Vitamin B1 (thiamine) - 0.029 Vitamin B2 (riboflavin) - 0.037 mg Niacin - 0.93 mg Folate - 36 mcg Pantothenic Acid - 0.397 mg Vitamin B6 - 0.043 mg Vitamin C - 30.2

		mg Zinc - 0.76 mg Also contains small amounts of other minerals.	mg Vitamin E - 1.68 mg Vitamin K - 28.5 mcg Contains some other vitamins in small amounts.
Blackcurrants	One cup of blackcurrants contains 1.57 grams of protein and 71 calories.	Potassium - 361 mg Phosphorus - 66 mg Magnesium - 27 mg Calcium - 62 mg Sodium - 2 mg Iron - 1.72 mg Manganese - 0.287 mg Copper - 0.096 mg Zinc - 0.3 mg Also contains small amounts of other minerals.	Vitamin A - 258 IU Vitamin B1 (thiamine) - 0.056 mg Vitamin B2 (riboflavin) - 0.056 mg Niacin - 0.336 mg Pantothenic Acid - 0.446 mg Vitamin B6 - 0.074 mg Vitamin C - 202.7 mg Vitamin E - 1.12 mg Contains some other vitamins in small amounts.
Blueberries	One cup of blueberries contains 1.1 grams of protein, 84 calories and 3.6 grams of dietary fiber.	Potassium - 114 mg Phosphorus - 18 mg Magnesium - 9 mg Calcium - 9 mg Sodium - 1 mg Iron - 0.41 mg Selenium 0.1 mcg Manganese - 0.497 mg Zinc - 0.24 mg Also contains small amounts of other minerals.	Vitamin A - 217 IU Vitamin B1 (thiamine) - 0.055 mg Vitamin B2 (riboflavin) - 0.061 mg Niacin - 0.08 mg Folate - 9 mcg Pantothenic Acid - 0.184 mg Vitamin B6 - 0.077 mg Vitamin C - 14.4 mg Vitamin E - 2.29 mg Vitamin K - 28.6 mcg Contains some other vitamins in small amounts.
Boysenberries	One cup of frozen boysenberries contains 1.45 grams of protein, 66 calories and	Potassium - 183 mg Phosphorus - 36 mg Magnesium - 21 mg Calcium - 36 mg	Vitamin A - 88 IU Vitamin B1 (thiamine) - 0.07 mg Vitamin B2 (riboflavin) - 0.049 mg

	7 grams of dietary fiber.	Sodium - 1 mg Iron - 1.12 mg Selenium 0.3 mcg Manganese - 0.722 mg Copper - 0.106 mg Zinc - 0.29 mg Also contains small amounts of other minerals.	Niacin - 1.012 mg Folate - 83 mcg Pantothenic Acid - 0.33 mg Vitamin B6 - 0.074 mg Vitamin C - 4.1 mg Vitamin E - 1.15 mg Vitamin K - 10.3 mcg Contains some other vitamins in small amounts.
Breadfruit	One cup of fresh breadfruit contains 2.35 grams of protein, 227 calories and 10.8 grams of dietary fiber.	Potassium - 1078 mg Phosphorus - 66 mg Magnesium - 55 mg Calcium - 37 mg Sodium - 4 mg Iron - 1.19 mg Selenium 1.3 mcg Manganese - 0.132 mg Copper - 0.185 mg Zinc - 0.26 mg Also contains small amounts of other minerals.	Vitamin B1 (thiamine) - 0.242 mg Vitamin B2 (riboflavin) - 0.066 mg Niacin - 1.98 mg Folate - 31 mcg Pantothenic Acid - 1.05 mg Vitamin B6 - 0.22 mg Vitamin C - 63.8 mg Vitamin E - 0.22 mg Vitamin K - 1.1 mcg Contains some other vitamins in small amounts.
Cantaloupe	One medium wedge (slice) of cantaloupe contains 0.58 grams of protein, 23 calories and 0.6 grams of dietary fiber.	Potassium - 184 mg Phosphorus - 10 mg Magnesium - 8 mg Calcium - 6 mg Sodium - 11 mg Iron - 0.14 mg Selenium 0.3 mcg Manganese - 0.028 mg Copper - 0.028 mg Zinc - 0.12 mg Also contains small amounts of other minerals.	Vitamin A - 2334 IU Vitamin B1 (thiamine) - 0.028 mg Vitamin B2 (riboflavin) - 0.013 mg Niacin - 0.506 mg Folate - 14 mcg Pantothenic Acid - 0.072 mg Vitamin B6 - 0.05 mg Vitamin C - 25.3 mg Vitamin E - 0.03 mg Vitamin K - 1.7 mcg Contains some other vitamins in small amounts.
Cherimoya	One cup of	Potassium - 459	Vitamin B1

	diced, fresh cherimoya contains 2.51 grams of protein, 120 calories and 4.8 grams of dietary fiber.	mg Phosphorus - 42 mg Magnesium - 27 mg Calcium - 16 mg Sodium - 11 mg Iron - 0.43 mg Manganese - 0.149 mg Copper - 0.11 mg Zinc - 0.26 mg Also contains small amounts of other minerals.	(thiamine) - 0.162 mg Vitamin B2 (riboflavin) - 0.21 mg Niacin - 1.03 mg Folate - 37 mcg Pantothenic Acid - 0.552 mg Vitamin B6 - 0.411 mg Vitamin C - 20.2 mg Vitamin A - 8 IU Vitamin E - 0.43 mg Contains some other vitamins in small amounts.
Cherries	One cup of fresh cherries, with pits, contains 1.46 grams of protein, 87 calories and 2.9 grams of dietary fiber.	Potassium - 306 mg Phosphorus - 29 mg Magnesium - 15 mg Calcium - 18 mg Iron - 0.5 mg Zinc - 0.1 mg Manganese - 0.097 mg Copper - 0.083 mg Also contains small amounts of other minerals.	Vitamin A - 88 IU Vitamin B1 (thiamine) - 0.037 mg Vitamin B2 (riboflavin) - 0.046 mg Niacin - 0.213 mg Folate - 6 mcg Pantothenic Acid - 0.275 mg Vitamin B6 - 0.068 mg Vitamin C - 9.7 mg Vitamin E - 0.1 mg Vitamin K - 2.9 mcg Contains some other vitamins in small amounts.
Chinese pear	One Chinese (Asian) pear, about 3 inches in diameter, contains 1.38 grams of protein, 116 calories and 9.9 grams of dietary fiber.	Potassium - 333 mg Phosphorus - 30 mg Magnesium - 22 mg Calcium - 11 mg Selenium 0.3 mcg Manganese - 0.165 mg Copper - 0.138 mg Zinc - 0.06 mg Also contains small amounts of other minerals.	Vitamin B1 (thiamine) - 0.025 mg Vitamin B2 (riboflavin) - 0.028 mg Niacin - 0.602 mg Folate - 22 mcg Pantothenic Acid - 0.193 mg Vitamin B6 - 0.06 mg Vitamin C - 10.4 mg Vitamin E - 0.33 mg Vitamin K - 12.4 mcg Contains some

			other vitamins in small amounts.
Cranberries	One cup of cranberries contains 0.39 grams of protein, 46 calories and 4.6 grams of dietary fiber.	Potassium - 85 mg Phosphorus - 13 mg Magnesium - 6 mg Calcium - 8 mg Sodium - 2 mg Iron - 0.25 mg Selenium 0.1 mcg Manganese - 0.36 mg Copper - 0.061 mg Zinc - 0.1 mg Also contains small amounts of other minerals.	Vitamin A - 60 IU Vitamin B1 (thiamine) - 0.012 mg Vitamin B2 (riboflavin) - 0.02 mg Niacin - 0.101 mg Folate - 1 mcg Pantothenic Acid - 0.295 mg Vitamin B6 - 0.057 mg Vitamin C - 13.3 mg Vitamin E - 1.2 mg Vitamin K - 5.1 mcg Contains some other vitamins in small amounts.
Figs	One large, fresh fig contains 0.48 grams of protein, 47 calories and 1.9 grams of dietary fiber.	Potassium - 148 mg Phosphorus - 9 mg Magnesium - 11 mg Calcium - 22 mg Sodium - 1 mg Iron - 0.24 mg Selenium 0.1 mcg Manganese - 0.082 mg Copper - 0.045 mg Zinc - 0.1 mg Also contains small amounts of other minerals.	Vitamin A - 91 IU Vitamin B1 (thiamine) - 0.038 mg Vitamin B2 (riboflavin) - 0.032 mg Niacin - 0.256 mg Folate - 4 mcg Pantothenic Acid - 0.192 mg Vitamin B6 - 0.072 mg Vitamin C - 1.3 mg Vitamin E - 0.07 mg Vitamin K - 3 mcg Contains some other vitamins in small amounts.
Gooseberries	One cup of gooseberries contains 1.32 grams of protein, 66 calories and over 6.5 grams of dietary fiber.	Potassium - 297 mg Phosphorus - 40 mg Magnesium - 15 mg Calcium - 38 mg Sodium - 2 mg Iron - 0.47 mg Selenium 0.9 mcg Manganese - 0.216 mg Copper - 0.105	Vitamin A - 435 IU Vitamin B1 (thiamine) - 0.06 mg Vitamin B2 (riboflavin) - 0.045 mg Niacin - 0.45 mg Folate - 9 mcg Pantothenic Acid - 0.429 mg Vitamin B6 - 0.12 mg Vitamin C - 41.5

		mg Zinc - 0.18 mg Also contains small amounts of other minerals.	mg Vitamin E - 0.56 mg Contains some other vitamins in small amounts.
Grapes	One cup of grapes contains 1.09 gram of protein, 104 calories and 1.4 grams of dietary fiber.	Potassium - 288 mg Phosphorus - 30 mg Magnesium - 11 mg Calcium - 15 mg Sodium - 3 mg Iron - 0.54 mg Selenium 0.2 mcg Manganese - 0.107 mg Copper - 0.192 mg Zinc - 0.11 mg Also contains small amounts of other minerals.	Vitamin A - 100 IU Vitamin B1 (thiamine) - 0.104 mg Vitamin B2 (riboflavin) - 0.106 mg Niacin - 0.284 mg Folate - 3 mcg Pantothenic Acid - 0.076 mg Vitamin B6 - 0.13 mg Vitamin C - 16.3 mg Vitamin E - 0.29 mg Vitamin K - 22 mcg Contains some other vitamins in small amounts.
Guava	One cup of fresh guava contains 4.21 grams of protein, 112 calories and 8.9 grams of dietary fiber.	Potassium - 688 mg Phosphorus - 66 mg Magnesium - 36 mg Calcium - 30 mg Sodium - 3 mg Iron - 0.43 mg Selenium 1 mcg Manganese - 0.247 mg Copper - 0.38 mg Zinc - 0.38 mg Also contains small amounts of other minerals.	Vitamin A - 1030 IU Vitamin B1 (thiamine) - 0.111 mg Vitamin B2 (riboflavin) - 0.066 mg Niacin - 1.789 mg Folate - 81 mcg Pantothenic Acid - 0.744 mg Vitamin B6 - 0.181 mg Vitamin C - 376.7 mg Vitamin E - 1.2 mg Vitamin K - 4.3 mcg Contains some other vitamins in small amounts.
Lemon	One lemon without peel contains 0.92 grams protein, 24 calories and 2.4 grams of dietary fiber.	Potassium - 116 mg Phosphorus - 13 mg Magnesium - 7 mg Calcium - 22 mg Sodium - 2 mg Iron - 0.5	Vitamin A - 18 IU Vitamin B1 (thiamine) - 0.034 mg Vitamin B2 (riboflavin) - 0.017 mg Niacin - 0.084 mg Folate - 9 mcg

		Selenium 0.3 mcg Manganese - 0.025 mg Copper - 0.031 mg Zinc - 0.05 mg Also contains small amounts of other minerals.	Pantothenic Acid - 0.16 mg Vitamin B6 - 0.067 mg Vitamin C - 44.5 mg Vitamin E - 0.13 mg Contains some other vitamins in small amounts.
Lime	One lime contains 0.47 grams of protein, 20 calories and 1.9 grams of dietary fiber.	Potassium - 68 mg Phosphorus - 12 mg Magnesium - 4 mg Calcium - 22 mg Sodium - 1 mg Iron - 0.4 mg Selenium 0.3 mcg Manganese - 0.005 mg Copper - 0.044 mg Zinc - 0.07 mg Also contains small amounts of other minerals.	Vitamin A - 34 IU Vitamin B1 (thiamine) - 0.02 mg Vitamin B2 (riboflavin) - 0.013 mg Niacin - 0.134 mg Folate - 5 mcg Pantothenic Acid - 0.145 mg Vitamin B6 - 0.029 mg Vitamin C - 19.5 mg Vitamin E - 0.15 mg Vitamin K - 0.4 mcg Contains some other vitamins in small amounts.
Loganberries	One cup of frozen loganberries contains 2.23 grams of protein, 81 calories and 7.8 grams of dietary fiber.	Potassium - 213 mg Phosphorus - 38 mg Magnesium - 31 mg Calcium - 38 mg Sodium - 1 mg Iron - 0.94 mg Selenium 0.3 mcg Manganese - 1.833 mg Copper - 0.172 mg Zinc - 0.5 mg Also contains small amounts of other minerals.	Vitamin A - 51 IU Vitamin B1 (thiamine) - 0.074 mg Vitamin B2 (riboflavin) - 0.05 mg Niacin - 1.235 mg Folate - 38 mcg Pantothenic Acid - 0.359 mg Vitamin B6 - 0.096 mg Vitamin C - 22.5 mg Vitamin E - 1.28 mg Vitamin K - 11.5 mcg Contains some other vitamins in small amounts.
Lychee	One cup of fresh lychees	Potassium - 325 mg	Vitamin B1 (thiamine) - 0.021

	contains 1.58 grams of protein, 125 calories and 2.5 grams of dietary fiber.	Phosphorus - 59 mg Magnesium - 19 mg Calcium - 10 mg Sodium - 2 mg Iron - 0.59 mg Selenium 1.1 mcg Manganese - 0.104 mg Copper - 0.281 mg Zinc - 0.13 mg Also contains small amounts of other minerals.	mg Vitamin B2 (riboflavin) - 0.123 mg Niacin - 1.146 mg Folate - 27 mcg Vitamin B6 - 0.19 mg Vitamin C - 135.8 mg Vitamin E - 0.13 mg Vitamin K - 0.08 mcg Contains some other vitamins in small amounts.
Mango 	One mango without peel contains 1.06 grams of protein, 135 calories and 3.7 grams of dietary fiber.	Potassium - 323 mg Phosphorus - 23 mg Magnesium - 19 mg Calcium - 21 mg Sodium - 4 mg Iron - 0.27 mg Selenium 1.2 mcg Manganese - 0.056 mg Copper - 0.228 mg Zinc - 0.08 mg Also contains small amounts of other minerals.	Vitamin A - 1584 IU Vitamin B1 (thiamine) - 0.12 mg Vitamin B2 (riboflavin) - 0.118 mg Niacin - 1.209 mg Folate - 29 mcg Pantothenic Acid - 0.331 mg Vitamin B6 - 0.227 mg Vitamin C - 57.3 mg Vitamin E - 2.32 mg Vitamin K - 8.7 mcg Contains some other vitamins in small amounts.
Mulberries 	One cup of fresh mulberries contains 2.02 grams of protein and 2.4 grams of dietary fiber.	Potassium - 272 mg Phosphorus - 53 mg Magnesium - 25 mg Calcium - 55 mg Sodium - 14 mg Iron - 2.59 mg Selenium 0.8 mcg Copper - 0.084 mg Zinc - 0.17 mg Also contains small amounts of other minerals.	Vitamin A - 35 IU Vitamin B1 (thiamine) - 0.041 mg Vitamin B2 (riboflavin) - 0.141 mg Niacin - 0.868 mg Folate - 8 mcg Vitamin B6 - 0.07 mg Vitamin C - 51 mg Vitamin E - 1.22 mg Vitamin K - 10.9 mcg Contains some other vitamins in small amounts.

Nectarine	One cup of sliced fresh nectarine contains 1.52 grams of protein, 63 calories and 2.4 grams of dietary fiber.	Potassium - 287 mg Phosphorus - 37 mg Magnesium - 13 mg Calcium - 9 mg Iron - 0.4 mg Manganese - 0.077 mg Copper - 0.123 mg Zinc - 0.24 mg Also contains small amounts of other minerals.	Vitamin A - 475 IU Vitamin B1 (thiamine) - 0.049 mg Vitamin B2 (riboflavin) - 0.039 mg Niacin - 1.609 mg Folate - 7 mcg Pantothenic Acid - 0.265 mg Vitamin B6 - 0.036 mg Vitamin C - 7.7 mg Vitamin E - 1.1 mg Vitamin K - 3.1 mcg Contains some other vitamins in small amounts.
Olives	One tablespoon of ripe olives contains 0.07 grams of protein, 10 calories and 0.3 grams of dietary fiber.	Potassium - 1 mg Calcium - 7 mg Sodium - 73 mg Iron - 0.28 mg Selenium 0.1 mcg Manganese - 0.002 mg Copper - 0.021 mg Zinc - 0.02 mg Also contains small amounts of other minerals.	Vitamin A - 34 IU Niacin - 0.003 mg Pantothenic Acid - 0.001 mg Vitamin B6 - 0.001 mg Vitamin C - 0.1 mg Vitamin E - 0.14 mg Vitamin K - 0.1 mcg Contains some other vitamins in small amounts.
Papaya	One cup of cubed fresh papaya contains 0.85 grams of protein, 55 calories and 2.5 grams of dietary fiber.	Potassium - 360 mg Phosphorus - 7 mg Magnesium - 14 mg Calcium - 34 mg Sodium - 4 mg Iron - 0.14 mg Selenium 0.8 mcg Zinc - 0.1 mg Manganese - 0.015 mg Copper - 0.022 mg Also contains small amounts of other minerals.	Vitamin A - 1532 IU Vitamin B1 (thiamine) - 0.038 mg Vitamin B2 (riboflavin) - 0.045 mg Niacin - 0.473 mg Folate - 53 mcg Pantothenic Acid - 0.305 mg Vitamin B6 - 0.027 mg Vitamin C - 86.5 mg Vitamin E - 1.02 mg Vitamin K - 3.6 mcg Contains some other vitamins in small amounts.
Passion fruit	One cup of	Potassium - 821	Vitamin A - 3002 IU

	fresh passion fruit contains 5.19 grams of protein, 229 calories and 24.5 grams of dietary fiber.	mg Phosphorus - 160 mg Magnesium - 68 mg Calcium - 28 mg Sodium - 66 mg Iron - 3.78 mg Selenium 1.4 mcg Copper - 0.203 mg Zinc - 0.24 mg Also contains small amounts of other minerals.	Vitamin B2 (riboflavin) - 0.307 mg Niacin - 3.54 mg Folate - 33 mcg Vitamin B6 - 0.236 mg Vitamin C - 70.8 mg Vitamin E - 0.05 mg Vitamin K - 1.7 mcg Contains some other vitamins in small amounts.
Peach 	One medium peach (with skin) contains 1.36 grams of protein, 58 calories and 2.2 grams dietary fiber.	Potassium - 285 mg Phosphorus - 30 mg Magnesium - 14 mg Calcium - 9 mg Iron - 0.38 mg Selenium 0.1 mcg Manganese - 0.091 mg Copper - 0.102 mg Zinc - 0.26 mg Also contains small amounts of other minerals.	Vitamin A - 489 IU Vitamin B1 (thiamine) - 0.036 mg Vitamin B2 (riboflavin) - 0.047 mg Niacin - 1.209 mg Folate - 6 mcg Pantothenic Acid - 0.229 mg Vitamin B6 - 0.037 mg Vitamin C - 9.9 mg Vitamin E - 1.09 mg Vitamin K - 3.9 mcg Contains some other vitamins in small amounts.
Pear 	One medium pear contains 0.68 grams of protein, 103 calories and 5.5 grams dietary fiber.	Potassium - 212 mg Phosphorus - 20 mg Magnesium - 12 mg Calcium -16 mg Sodium - 2 mg Iron - 0.3 mg Selenium 0.2 mcg Manganese - 0.087 mg Copper - 0.146 mg Zinc - 0.18 mg Also contains small amounts of other minerals.	Vitamin A - 41 IU Vitamin B1 (thiamine) - 0.021 mg Vitamin B2 (riboflavin) - 0.045 mg Niacin - 0.279 mg Folate - 12 mcg Pantothenic Acid - 0.085 mg Vitamin B6 - 0.05 mg Vitamin C - 7.5 mg Vitamin E - 0.21 mg Vitamin K - 8 mcg Contains some other vitamins in small amounts.

Persimmon	One fresh persimmon contains 0.2 grams of protein and 32 calories.	Potassium - 78 mg Phosphorus - 6 mg Calcium - 7 mg Iron - 0.62 mg Also contains small amounts of other minerals.	Vitamin C - 16.5 mg Contains some other vitamins in small amounts.
Plum	One cup of sliced, fresh plums contains 1.15 grams of protein, 76 calories and 2.3 grams dietary fiber.	Potassium - 259 mg Phosphorus - 26 mg Magnesium - 12 mg Calcium - 10 mg Iron - 0.28 mg Manganese - 0.086 mg Copper - 0.094 mg Zinc - 0.17 mg Also contains small amounts of other minerals.	Vitamin A - 569 IU Vitamin B1 (thiamine) - 0.046 mg Vitamin B2 (riboflavin) - 0.043 mg Niacin - 0.688 mg Folate - 8 mcg Pantothenic Acid - 0.223 mg Vitamin B6 - 0.048 mg Vitamin C - 15.7 mg Vitamin E - 0.43 mg Vitamin K - 10.6 mcg Contains some other vitamins in small amounts.
Pomegranate	One fresh pomegranate contains 4.71 grams of protein, 234 calories and 11.3 grams dietary fiber.	Potassium - 666 mg Phosphorus - 102 mg Magnesium - 34 mg Calcium - 28 mg Sodium - 8 mg Iron - 0.85 mg Selenium 1.4 mcg Manganese - 0.336 mg Copper - 0.446 mg Zinc - 0.99 mg Also contains small amounts of other minerals.	Vitamin B1 (thiamine) - 0.189 mg Vitamin B2 (riboflavin) - 0.149 mg Niacin - 0.826 mg Folate - 107 mcg Pantothenic Acid - 1.063 mg Vitamin B6 - 0.211 mg Vitamin C - 28.8 mg Vitamin E - 1.69 mg Vitamin K - 46.2 mcg Contains some other vitamins in small amounts.
Prickly Pear	One cup of raw prickly pears contains 1.09	Potassium - 328 mg Phosphorus - 36 mg	Vitamin A - 64 IU Vitamin B1 (thiamine) - 0.021 mg

	grams of protein, 61 calories and 5.4 grams dietary fiber.	Magnesium - 127 mg Calcium - 83 mg Sodium - 7 mg Iron - 0.45 mg Selenium 0.9 mcg Copper - 0.119 mg Zinc - 0.18 mg Also contains small amounts of other minerals.	Vitamin B2 (riboflavin) - 0.089 mg Niacin - 0.685 mg Vitamin B6 - 0.089 mg Folate - 9 mcg Vitamin C - 20.9 mg Contains some other vitamins in small amounts.
Star fruit aka Carambola 	One cup of fresh star fruit contains 1.37 grams of protein, 41 calories and 3.7 grams dietary fiber.	Potassium - 176 mg Phosphorus - 16 mg Magnesium - 13 mg Calcium - 4 mg Sodium - 3 mg Iron - 0.11 mg Selenium 0.8 mcg Manganese - 0.049 mg Copper - 0.181 mg Zinc - 0.16 mg Also contains small amounts of other minerals.	Vitamin A - 81 IU Vitamin B1 (thiamine) - 0.018 mg Vitamin B2 (riboflavin) - 0.021 mg Niacin - 0.484 mg Folate - 16 mcg Pantothenic Acid - 0.516 mg Vitamin B6 - 0.022 mg Vitamin C - 45.4 mg Vitamin E - 0.2 mg Contains some other vitamins in small amounts.
Watermelon 	I medium wedge (slice) of watermelon (about 2 cups edible portion) contains 1.74 grams of protein, 86 calories and 1.1 grams of dietary fiber.	Potassium - 320 mg Phosphorus - 31 mg Magnesium - 29 mg Calcium - 20 mg Sodium - 3 mg Iron - 0.69 mg Selenium 1.1 mcg Manganese - 0.109 mg Copper - 0.12 mg Zinc - 0.29 mg Also contains small amounts of other minerals.	Vitamin A - 1627 IU Vitamin B1 (thiamine) - 0.094 mg Vitamin B2 (riboflavin) - 0.06 mg Niacin - 0.509 mg Folate - 9 mcg Pantothenic Acid - 0.632 mg Vitamin B6 - 0.129 mg Vitamin C - 23.2 mg Vitamin E - 0.14 mg Vitamin K - 0.3 mcg Contains some other vitamins in small amounts.

Chapter 10

The Secrets of a Cancer-Free People

*There are two ways to live **your life**. One is as though nothing is a miracle. The other is as **though everything is a miracle** –*

Albert Einstein.

How would you like to live in a land where cancer does not exist? A land where an optometrist discovers to his amazement that everyone has perfect 20-20 vision? A land where cardiologists cannot find a single trace of **coronary heart disease**? How would you like to live in a land where no one ever gets **heart ailments, cancer, arthritis, high blood pressure, diabetes, tuberculosis, hay fever, asthma, liver trouble, gall bladder trouble, constipation, ulcers, appendicitis, and gout**? A land where it is not unusual for men and women to enjoy vigorous life at the age of 100 or 120?

Does such an apparently magical place like that actually exist on our beautiful planet Earth?

It exists! A tiny, little hidden region in the Himalaya mountains, a place called Hunza in the high passes between the borders of China, Russia, India and Pakistan. Would you like to experience this life? You'll see how special this lifestyle is when you ask yourself a few questions:

1. Are you willing to live 20,000 feet up in the mountains, almost completely out of touch with the rest of the world?

2. Are you ready to go outside in every kind of weather to tend your small mountainside garden, while keeping your ears open for an impending avalanche?

3. Are you prepared to give up not only every luxury of civilization, but even reading, writing and Internet access?

Quite major change requirements, right? At the same time if you want the benefits of the pure air that whips by the icy cathedrals of the Himalayan Mountains, the pure water that dances down from glaciers formed at 25,000 feet, and the mental and spiritual peace that comes from living in a land where there is no crime, taxes, social striving or generation gaps, no banks or stores-in fact-no money- where could you possibly find it outside of Hunza?

But don't give up! Not yet, because there is still one more question to be answered. Which is: **Are you prepared to eat the kind of food the Hunza people eat**? If you are, then you can rightfully expect to give yourself at least a useful measure of the **super health** and **resistance** to degenerative disease, which the Hunzakuts have enjoyed for more than 2,000 years.

You are wondering what kind of exotic, ill-tasting foods do these Hunza people eat? It may sound very strange to you, actually everything the Hunzakuts eat is delectable to the western palate, and is readily available in the United States and Europe - at least if you shopping horizons do not begin and end at the typical supermarket.

Not only is the Hunza diet not exotic; there's really nothing terribly mysterious about its health-promoting qualities. Everything we know about food and health, gathered both from clinical studies and the observation of scientists who have traveled throughout the world observing dietary practices and their relationship to health, tells us that it is to be expected that the Hunza diet will go a long way towards dramatically improving the total health of anyone, anywhere. The Hunza story is only one of the more dramatic examples of the miraculous health produced by a diet of fresh, natural unprocessed and unadulterated food.

Are the People of Hunza that Healthy?

Maybe you're wondering: are the Hunzas really all that healthy? That was the question on the mind of cardiologists Dr. Paul D. White and Dr. Edward G. Toomey, who made the difficult trip up the mountain paths to Hunza, toting along with them a portable, battery-operated electrocardiograph. In the American Heart Journal for December 1964, the doctors say they used the equipment to study 25 Hunza men, who were, "on fairly good evidence, between 90 and 110 years old." Blood pressure and cholesterol levels were also tested. They reported that not one of these men showed a single sign of coronary heart disease, high blood pressure or high cholesterol.

An optometrist, Dr. Allen E. Banik, also made the journey to Hunza to see himself if the people were as healthy as they were reputed to be, and published his report in Hunza Land (Whitethorn Publishing Co., 1960). "It wasn't long before I discovered that everything that I had read about perpetual life and health in this tiny country is true, "Dr. Banik declared." I examined the eyes of some of Hunza's oldest citizens and found them to be perfect."

Beyond more freedom from disease, the positive side of Hunza health has startled many observers. Dr. Banik, for example, relates that "many Hunza people are so strong that in the winter they exercise by breaking holes in the ice-covered streams and take a swim down under the ice." Other intrepid visitors who have been there report their amazement at seeing men 80, 90, and 100 years old repairing the always-crumbling rocky roads, and lifting large stones and boulders to repair the retaining walls around their terrace gardens. The oldsters think nothing of playing a competitive game of volleyball in the hot sun against men 50 years their junior, and even take part in wild games of polo that are so violent they would make an ice hockey fan shudder.

The energy and endurance of the Hunzakuts can probably be credited as much to what they don't eat as what they do eat. First of all, they don't eat a great deal of anything. The United States Department of Agriculture estimates that the average daily food intake for Americans of all ages amounts to 3,300 calories, with 100 grams of protein, 157 grams of fat and 380 grams of carbohydrates, In contrast, studies by Pakistani doctors show that adult males of Hunza consume a little more than 1.900 calories daily, with only 50 grams of protein, 36 grams of healthy fat, and 354 grams of carbohydrates. Both the **protein** and **fat** are **largely of**

vegetable origin (Dr. Alexander Leaf, National Geographic, January, 1973).

That amounts to just half the protein, one-third the fat, but about the same amount of carbohydrates that we eat. Of course, the carbohydrate that the Hunzakuts eat is **undefined** or **complex carbohydrate** found in **fruits, vegetables** and **grains**, while we largely eat our carbohydrates in the form of nutrition like **white sugar** and **refined flour**.

Needless to say, the Hunzakuts eat **no processed food**. Everything is as fresh as it can possibly be. The only "processing" consists of **drying** certain fresh fruits in the sun. No chemicals or artificial fertilizers are used in their gardens. In fact, it is against the law of Hunza to spray gardens with **pesticides.** Renee Taylor, in her book, Hunza Health Secrets (Prentice-Hall 1964) says that the Mir, or ruler of Hunza, was recently instructed by Pakistani authorities to spray the orchards of Hunza with pesticide, to protect them from an expected invasion of insects. But the Hunzas would have none of it. They refused to use the **toxic pesticide**, and instead sprayed their trees with a mixture of **water** and **ashes**, which **adequately** protected the trees without poisoning the fruit and the entire environment. **In a word, the Hunzas eat as they live-organically.**

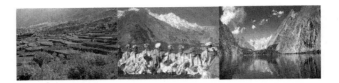

Apricots Are Hunza's Gold

Of all their organically grown food, perhaps their favorite, and one of their dietary mainstays, is the **apricot**. Apricot orchards are seen everywhere in Hunza, and a family's economic stability is measured by the number of trees they have under cultivation.

They eat their apricots **fresh in season**, and dry a great deal more in the sun for eating throughout the long cold winter. They puree the dried apricots and mix them with snow to make ice cream. Like their apricot jam, this ice cream needs no sugar because the apricots are so sweet naturally. But that is only the beginning.

The Hunzas cut the pits from the fruits, crack them, remove and eat the almond-like nuts. The women hand-grind these kernels with stone mortars, then squeeze the meal between a hand stone and a flat rock to **express the oil**. The oil is used in cooking, for fuel, as a salad dressing on fresh garden greens, and even as a **facial lotion** (Renee Taylor says Hunza women have beautiful complexions).

The Apricot Kernels Anti-Cancer Theory

Do these kernels have important protective powers, which in some way play an important role in the extraordinary health and longevity of the Hunza people? The **evidence** suggests they very well might. Cancer and arthritis are both very rare among the Taos (New Mexico) Pueblo Indians. Their traditional beverages are made from the group **kernels of cherries, peaches and apricots**.

Dr. Robert G. Houston told PREVENTION that he enjoyed this beverage when he was in New Mexico gathering material for a book dealing with blender shakes based on an Indian recipe. Into a glass of juice, he mixed freshly ground apricot kernels (1/4 of an ounce or two dozen kernels), which had been roasted for 10 minutes at 300 F. It is vitally important to roast the kernels first. Houston points out, "in order to ensure safety when you are using the pits in such quantities." Roasting destroys enzymes which could upset your stomach if you eat too many at on time. In any event the drink was so delicious that Houston kept having it daily. On the third day of drinking this concoction, Houston says that a funny thing happened. Two little benign skin growths on his arm, which formerly were pink, had turned brown. The next day, he noticed that the growths were black and shriveled. On the seventh morning, the smaller more recent growths had **vanished completely and the larger one about the size of a grain of rice had simply fallen off.**

Dr. Houston says that two of his friends have since tried the apricot shakes and report similar elimination of benign skin growths in one or two weeks. "Some foods, especially the kernels of certain fruits and grains, contain elements known as the nitrilosides also known as amygdalin or **Vitamin B 17**" says Dr. Ernst T. Krebs, Jr., biochemist and co-discoverer of Laetrile, a controversial cancer treatment (Laetrile is the proprietary name for one nitriloside). Nitrilosides, says Dr. Krebs, are non-toxic water-soluble, accessory food factors found in abundance in the **seeds** of almost **all fruits**. They are also found in over **100** other plants.

There are other common foods (all seeds), which provide a goodly supply of this protective factor, for example Hunzakuts eat in abundance **millet** and **buckwheat**. Lentils, beans and alfalfa, when sprouted, provide 50 times more nitrilosides than does the mature plant, Dr. Krebs points out. And the Hunzas, as you might expect, sprout all of their seeds, as well as using them in other ways. Since other essential protective elements are increased in the sprouting of such seeds, young sprouts are excellent foods, which give us more life-giving values than most of us realize.

Genesis 1:29

Then God said, *"I give you every seed-bearing plant on the face of the whole earth and every tree that has fruit with seed in it. They will be yours for food."*

Vitamin B 17

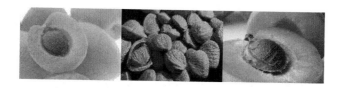

The Hunza people always crack open the kernel and eat the **seed.** The apricot seed contains Vitamin B17. Vitamin B17 is the **anticancer vitamin**. Some researchers have found that cancer and sickle cell anemia are caused by a **deficiency of vitamin B17**. Just as scurvy is caused by a deficiency of vitamin C, pernicious anemia is due to a deficiency of vitamin B12 and folic acid, and pellagra is caused by a deficiency of vitamin B3.

Vitamin B17 kills cancer cells without harming normal cells, **making it nature's chemotherapy**.

Various documents from the oldest civilisations such as Egypt at the time of the Pharaohs and from China 2,500 years before Christ mention the therapeutic use of derivatives of **bitter almonds**. Egyptian papyri from 5,000 years ago mention the use of "aqua amigdalorum" for the treatment of some **tumours** of the skin. But the systematised study of Vitamin B-17 really did not begin until the first half of the past century, when the chemist Bohn discovered in 1802 that during the distillation of the water from bitter almonds hydrocyanic acid was released. Soon many researchers became interested in analysing this extract, which they called AMYGDALIN (from amygdala = almond).

Vitamin B17 As a Preventative

According to Dr. Krebs, the basic concept is that sufficient daily B-17 may be obtained by following either of two suggestions:

First, eating all the B-17-containing food and seeds, but not eating more of the seeds by themselves than you would be eating if you ate them in the whole fruit. Example: if you eat **three apples** a day, **the seeds in the three apples are sufficient B-17**. You would never eat a pound of apple seeds.

Second, one peach or apricot kernel per 10 lbs. of body weight is believed to be more than sufficient as a normal safeguard in cancer prevention and chemotherapy help, although precise numbers may vary from person to person in accordance with individual metabolism and dietary habits. A 170-lb man, for example, might consume up to 17 apricots or peach kernels per day and receive a biologically reasonable amount of Vitamin B-17.

And two important notes: Certainly, you can consume too much of anything. Too many kernels or seeds, for example, can be expected to produce unpleasant side effects. **Too much is too much!**

High concentrations of B-17 are obtained by eating the natural foods in their raw or sprouting stage.

So how does B17 kill cancer cells?

Firstly, we need to understand that our bodies use several enzymes to perform many tasks. Our body has one particular enzyme called Rhodanese, which is found in large quantities throughout the body but **is not present wherever there are cancer cells.** Yet, wherever you find cancer in the body, you find another enzyme called Beta-Glucosidase. So, we have the enzyme Rhodanese found everywhere in the body except at the cancer cells, and we have the enzyme Beta-Glucosidase found in very large quantities only at the cancer cell but not found anywhere else in the body. If there is no cancer in the body there is no enzyme Beta-Glucosidase.

Now the following is what scares most people. You see Vitamin B17 is made up of 2 parts glucose, 1 part Hydrogen Cyanide and 1 part Benzaldehyde (analgesic/painkiller). So it is very important you understand the following:

When **B17** is introduced to the body, the enzyme called Rhodanese breaks it down. The Rhodanese breaks the Hydrogen Cyanide and Benzaldehyde down into 2 by-products, Thiocyanate and Benzoic acid, which are beneficial in **nourishing healthy cells** and forms the metabolic pool production for vitamin B12. Any excess of these by-products is expelled in normal fashion from the body via urine. Vitamin B17 passes through your body and does not last longer than 80 minutes inside your body as a result of the Rhodanese breaking it down. (Hydrogen Cyanide has been proven to be chemically inert and non-toxic when taken as food or refined pharmaceutical such as laetrile. Sugar has been shown to be 20 times more toxic than B17 - see good & bad cyanide).

AND HERE IS THE BEST PART:

When the B17 comes into contact with **cancer cells**, there is no Rhodanese to break it down and neutralize it but instead, only the enzyme Beta-Glucosidase is present in very large quantities. When B17 and Beta-Glucosidase come into contact with each other, a chemical reaction occurs and the Hydrogen Cyanide and Benzaldehyde combine synergistically to produce a poison, which destroys and kills the cancer cells. This whole process is known as selective toxicity. Only the cancer cells are specifically targeted and destroyed. See the diagram below.

Here is an illustration of how Vitamin B17 Kills Cancer. It has been proven to work by the some of the top cancer specialists in the world.

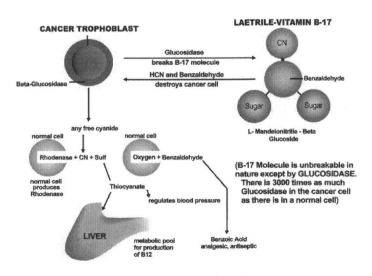

The best as you know is to have everything in moderation, and we have to apply this rule here. I would recommend you take up to 5 apricot kernels a day plus the amount of apple seeds you can find in 2-3 apples and have the variety of food that contains Vitamin B 17 like spinach, alfalfa, beans etc. In the chart below you can see the food that is the most rich in B 17. The best way is to have variety of recommended food every day, that way you get the most nutrients and heal, **alkalize** and **detox** your body as quick as possible.

Vitamin B17 and foods that contain it

Vitamin B17 or Laetrile appears in abundance in untamed nature. Because B17 is bitter to the taste, in man's attempt to improve tastes and flavors for his own pleasure, he has eliminated bitter substances like B17 by selection and crossbreeding.

As a general rule, many of the foods that have been domesticated still contain the vitamin B17 in that part not eaten by modern man, such as the seeds in apricots as you know already.

Listed below is an evaluation of some of the more common foods. Keep in mind that these are averages only and that specimens vary widely depending on variety, locale, soil, and climate.

All fruits that are listed below should be organically grown and ripe.

Foods	Low content (below 100 mgs nitriloside per 100 grams food)	Medium content (above 100 mgs nitriloside per 100 grams food)	High content (above 100 mgs nitriloside per 100 grams food)
Fruits	Domestic blackberry, market cranberry	Boysenberry, currant, elderberry (medium to high), gooseberry, huckleberry loganberry, mulberry, quince, raspberry	Wild blackberry, choke cherry, wild crab-apple, Swedish (lignon) cranberry
Seeds		Buckwheat, flax, millet,	Apple seed, apricot seed, cherry seed, nectarine seed, peach seed, pear seeds, plum seed, prune seed, squash seeds
Beans	Black, black-eyed peas, garbanzo (low to	Lentils, Burma lima, mung (medium to high)	Fava

	medium), green pea, kidney (low to medium), U.S. lima, shell		
Leaves	Beet tops, spinach, water cress		Alfalfa, eucalyptus,
Nuts (raw)	Cashew	Macadamia (medium to high)	Bitter almond
Sprouts		Alfalfa, fava, garbanzo, mung	Bamboo
Tubers	Sweet potato, yams		Cassava

Chapter 11

Using Detoxification & Purification Techniques

*"**Understanding** is the **first step** to **acceptance**, and only with **acceptance** can there be **recovery**."*

J.K. Rowling

Why is detoxification of your body important?

Toxic agents and substances are everywhere in our world. The food we eat, the air we breathe, the household cleaners we spray, and the electronics we use on a daily basis. However, toxic free radicals are formed in the human body too. Stress hormones, emotional disturbances, anxiety and negative emotions all create free radicals as well. Living without toxic build up is virtually impossible, which is why our body has built in mechanisms to deal with toxic overload. Crying, sweating, urination and defecation are all natural protocols employed by the body to rid itself of toxins.

Despite overwhelming advancements in medical care our society is sicker than ever. We may be living longer, but we're riddled with illness and disease. Nearly all sickness in industrialized countries is due to toxic build up in the body. Often times toxins bind to sex hormones or thyroid hormones, which slows metabolism, causing weight gain. Additionally, toxins are stored in fat cells, also contributing to excess weight. Cardiovascular disease, cancer, polycystic ovarian syndrome, infertility, gastroesophageal reflux disease, fatty liver, gallstones, osteoarthritis, stroke, lower back pain, headaches, carpal tunnel syndrome, dementia, asthma and depression are just some of the illnesses associated with obesity.

Because toxins affect both the structure and function of cells, they cause a myriad of health problems in their own right. Chronic fatigue, fibromyalgia, autoimmune disorders like multiple sclerosis and lupus, migraines, premature aging, digestive problems like constipation, diarrhoea or bloating, skin conditions, aches and pains, PMS and food allergies or intolerances are all the result of toxic build up in the body.

Detoxification is so important because it can literally reverse the symptoms of illness and change your life. There are many different types of detoxification protocols and it is important to find one that works well for you. The liver, small intestine, kidneys, and colon are the major organs involved in the body's detoxification system. However, when employing any type of cleanse (like a juice cleanse, liver and gallbladder cleanse, elimination diet, heavy metal cleanse, etc.) it is important to first cleanse the kidneys and colon, as these two eliminative organs are responsible for carrying toxic waste out of the body. If they aren't cleared of blockages, you can end up with even more toxic build up, as the toxins that are being expelled have nowhere to go. Herbal formulas are especially good at cleansing the kidneys. Colon hydrotherapy, enemas and Epsom salt cleanses are all excellent way to cleanse the colon.

As a nutritionist though, I feel compelled to reiterate that **juice cleansing** is an absolutely wonderful way to thoroughly cleanse your entire body. Juice cleansing regimens can actually help you to lose unwanted fat, boost your mental clarity, improve the state of your skin, regulate digestion, and, most important, **remove toxins** from your system, and which is so critical in the case of those undergoing chemotherapy or radiation. As you do not have to chew and break down food when consuming juices, your digestive system is given a rest which allows time for your system to repair and rejuvenate. Juicing your food floods your body with **live enzymes** and an **abundance of antioxidants** that help not only neutralize free radicals but also strengthen and support the immune system, reduce blood pressure, improve sleep, concentration and memory, improve circulation and increase energy. Antioxidants even have anti-aging properties! They are literally a life-changing miracle food, and juice cleansing is an excellent way to inundate your system with them.

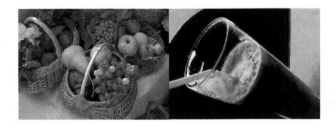

I am now confident of providing you with a holistic summary of the knowledge and suggestions passed on to you through the pages of my book:

1. Always alkalize your system by eliminating the food that contains too much acidity from your diet and include **Wheatgrass fresh juice** on its own or combined with other organically grown **fruit** or **vegetable** juices according to your taste. It is necessary to remove excess **acidity** and **toxic chemicals** from the body before health can be restored. To remove excess acidity from the tissues it is necessary to build up a reserve of alkalinity through an **alkaline (vegetarian) diet**, supplemented with **fresh fruit and vegetable juices** and **alkaline minerals**. Then this alkalinity must be moved around the body by any technique that works, such as exercise, massage, yoga, manual lymph drainage, etc. Vigorous **exercise** such as on the rebound mini-trampoline is reported to increase lymph flow by 15 to 30 times.

2. Avoid, at any cost, all dairy products including milk, cheese, yogurt, cream and ice cream with the one exception of organic butter in small quantities. Include delicious versions of organic cereals and nuts based "milk" drinks such as Almond Milk, Brown Rice Milk, Hazelnut Milk, Oat Milk, Quinoa Milk, etc. My personal favourites are hazelnut and almond milk.

3. The digestive system requires a rest periodically, even if just one day each week. Restricting the quantity of food consumed gives the system an opportunity to cleanse itself. The consumption of **fresh juices** made from **organically grown fruits and vegetables** during this time of reduced food consumption provides **alkalinity** to neutralize the acid wastes released from the tissues. It is important to understand that the doctors are not recommending "fasting" in the sense that you consume nothing but water. Rather they are recommending a liquid diet of fresh juices for a brief period (Diamond, pages 63, 341-42, 955).

4. Most people don't drink enough fluids every day and are chronically **dehydrated** without realizing it. We usually tend to drink liquids when feeling thirsty and this is already a critical stage for the body by then. As a result, the kidneys are quite overworked. A lot of people think that the more fluid they drink the more the kidneys must work to remove it. However, what is difficult for kidneys is to remove waste. Removing fluid is easy for the kidneys. The reason for this is the "**concentration gradient**". When people drink half the necessary amount of fluid, then waste in the urine is twice as concentrated. It is concentrating the waste that is difficult for the kidneys, because the kidneys need to overcome osmotic pressure that wants to equalize concentrations on both sides of the membrane. Healthy kidneys can achieve a concentration gradient of about 3:1. If you drink twice as much fluid then the wastes are diluted by half, allowing the kidneys to remove twice as much waste. **So drink more fluids and help the kidneys do their job.**

Up to 60% of the human body is water, the brain is composed of 70% water, and the lungs are nearly 90% water. Lean muscle tissue contains about 75% water by weight, body fat contains 10% water and bone has 22% water. About 83% of our blood is water, which helps digest our food, transport waste, and control body temperature. Each day the human body must replace 2.4 liters of water, some through drinking and the rest taken by the body from the foods eaten.

As was mentioned above, note that it is not good for your digestion to drink water less than 15 min before meals and not sooner than 40-45 min after meals.

5. An **alkaline condition** in the body increases zeta potential. Zeta potential is a measure of the electrical force that exists between atoms, molecules, particles, cells, etc., in a fluid. Zeta potential's strength determines the amount of nutrients and wastes that your blood and lymph can carry. Increasing the electrical force in the blood and lymph allows the fluid to dissolve and hold more nutrients, as a result releasing more waste. In this way, more nutrients can be carried throughout your body and **accumulated deposits of waste can be removed.** Aluminium (from food additives, cooking utensils, municipal drinking water, vaccines, drugs, etc.) destroys zeta potential.

Municipal (tap) drinking water contains chlorine. Chlorine has been used to disinfect our drinking water because it controls the growth of such unwelcome bacteria as Ecoli and Giardia. You have to be careful though when drinking tap water. Research has shown that long-term exposure to chlorine leads to the production of free radicals within the body. Free radicals as you know from above are carcinogenic, and cause tremendous damage to our cells.

The risk of developing cancer is 93% higher in people who drink or are otherwise exposed to chlorinated water.

How To Eliminate Chlorine in Water

- Consider a water purification system for your home. It will help to eliminate toxins before the water is used to cook, clean, shower and bathe.

- Use water filters in sinks and bathtubs. Water filters are an excellent way to ensure that your family is protected against the harmful effects of chlorine exposure.

- After you are exposed to chlorine, you should cleanse your body immediately. Use organic or all-natural soaps and detergents, as these are better for your skin. There are many kinds of soaps available that are not toxic.

Always drink purified water. Even better is oxygenated purified water, which provides added oxygen to your body.

6. Bile is an important avenue for detoxification of the body. It is a liquid produced by the **liver** and stored in the gallbladder until we eat a meal, and then it flows into the small intestine where it digests fats. Liver removes toxic chemicals from the blood, which flow out of the body via the bile and digestive tract. When the body produces more bile, the digestion improves and **more toxins** can be excreted via the bile. Inadequate bile flow allows toxins to build up in the body and results in liver disease, immune responses (allergies), skin problems, damaged arteries, arterial plaque, high blood pressure, chronic inflammation, arthritis, oedema (fluid build up), and cancer.

An **acid condition** in the body **causes bile to thicken**, eventually resulting in gallstones. Again you see the importance of an alkaline condition in the body, resulting in the bile to flow. Foods that help **increase bile** production and flow include **artichoke, lecithin, turmeric, and the herb milk thistle**.

Adequate bile is also needed for the body to digest and absorb fat-soluble vitamins and essential fatty acids.

7. Read the ingredients of all products you buy and make sure there are **no** sugar, soy, soybean oil, canola oil, bleached or unbleached wheat flower, soy flower, high fructose corn syrup (HFCS), corn syrup, trans fat, MSG, Aspartame, artificial sweeteners or dairy products.

8. Cook food using only coconut oil or virgin olive oil. Steam food rather than boiling when possible.

9. Steam bath and sauna are very helpful ways to purify the body through excessive sweating which removes toxic chemicals, and also because "**cancer cells die at temperatures between 104°F to 105.8°F** "(Diamond, page 996), whereas healthy cells survive.

Organic foods

As you noticed earlier in my book I emphasized the benefit of selecting organically grown foods. The explanation of this recommendation is quite simple. I would like you to understand in more detail the process of growing organic products and as a result the difference between organic products and conventional products.

Conventional vs. organic farming

The word "organic" refers to the way farmers grow and process agricultural products, such as fruits, vegetables, grains, fish, meat, etc. Organic farming practices are designed to encourage soil and water conservation and reduce pollution. Farmers who grow organic produce and meat don't use conventional methods to fertilize, control weeds or prevent livestock disease. For example, rather than using chemical weed killers, organic farmers may conduct more sophisticated crop rotations and spread mulch or manure to keep weeds at bay.

Here are some key differences between conventional farming and organic farming:

Conventional	Organic
Apply chemical fertilizers to promote plant growth.	Apply natural fertilizers, such as manure or compost, to feed soil and plants.
Spray synthetic insecticides to reduce pests and disease.	Spray pesticides from natural sources; use beneficial insects and birds, mating disruption or traps to reduce pests and disease.
Use synthetic herbicides to manage weeds.	Use environmentally generated plant-killing compounds; rotate crops, till, hand weed or mulch to manage weeds.
Give animals antibiotics, growth hormones and medications	Give animals organic feed and allow them access to the outdoors. Use preventive measures

to prevent disease and spur growth.	— such as rotational grazing, a balanced diet and clean housing — to help minimize disease.

The choice is yours! We are helping your body to detoxify, nourish, strength and heal itself with all available sources, and the right decision here is quite obvious.

More on Detoxification

A great choice for you will be to take Artichoke supplements or eat as a vegetable.

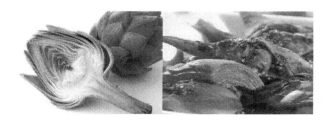

The Globe Artichoke is much valued at the table as a nutritious vegetable, but it is also an important aid to digestion and has been used to prevent arteriosclerosis. Artichoke extracts are said to be helpful for **kidney**, **gallbladder** and **liver insufficiency**, postoperative anaemia; and in some countries, Artichoke is considered a fine aphrodisiac.

Beneficial Uses:

The Artichoke has been used as an aid to good digestion and a means to improve **liver health**. Due to its cynarin content, it stimulates the **flow of bile from the liver into the intestines**, assisting the body in blood fat metabolism. Artichoke extracts are commercially available in Germany and Switzerland as a remedy for indigestion and in the U.K. as over-the-counter digestive supplements. The **cynarin compound**, which is found in the leaves, stimulates the **gallbladder** and **improves liver function**. Artichoke has been used traditionally and in alternative medicine for treating dyspepsia, indigestion, nausea, flatulence, as well as liver and gallbladder ailments, including jaundice and hepatitis.

By helping the body to metabolize blood fat, the cynarin content in Artichoke is also believed to reduce blood lipids, serum cholesterol and triglyceride levels and is thought to be helpful in controlling arteriosclerosis.

In 2008, U.K. research confirmed that Artichoke leaf extract could reduce cholesterol levels in healthy adults. The studies determined that when Artichoke leaf extract was administered to otherwise healthy adults with raised cholesterol, levels dropped 6%.

Highly nutritious Artichoke is considered a diuretic, **promoting the flow of urine and appears to be effective in improving kidney function.** Artichoke is also frequently used to relieve **excess water weight** and peripheral oedema, a condition in which the peripheral body tissues contain an excessive amount of tissue fluid.

Other qualities attributed to Artichoke use include hypoglycaemic activity that may assist in **lowering blood glucose levels**. Artichoke has had traditional uses in USA and Spain for treating **diabetes**.

It is one of the world's oldest cultivated vegetables, grown by the Greeks and Romans at the height of their power and used for **food** and **medicine**. In ancient Greek mythology, the god Zeus was said to love the Globe Artichoke, which gave rise to its nickname "Vegetable of the Gods."

Artichoke **leaves**, **flower heads** and **root** are used **medicinally**, and the leaves are cut just before flowering for use fresh or dried in liquid extracts, syrups and capsules. The French have long used Artichoke juice as a **liver tonic**, because of the herb's abilities to **break down fat** and improve **bile flow**.

Artichoke leaves contain a wide number of active constituents, including **cynarin** and **cholorogenic acid**, **flavonoids**, protein, **amino acids**, **calcium**, **phosphorus**, **potassium**, **folic acid**, **vitamin C, niacin, thiamine**, trace minerals and carotenoids.

Recommended Dosage:
Take two (2) capsules, two (2) times each day with water at mealtimes.

Contraindications:

Artichoke is not recommended for those who are allergic to Artichokes or other members of the *composites* (daisy) family. At the recommended amount and according to the German Commission E Monograph, there are no known side effects or drug interactions. **Those who have any obstruction of the bile duct (gallstones) should not take Artichoke.**

I would highly recommend, if you have the means and time to invest in a treatment of your body, mind and spirit by visiting, for a week or two, the Optimum Health Institute (OHI) or a similar establishment.

OHI has two locations, one in Texas and the other one in San Diego, California. OHI can offer you excellent programs for detoxification, cleansing and body nourishment as well as your mind and spirit.

OHI HOLISTIC HEALING PROGRAM:

In Optimum Health Institute's holistic healing program, participants cleanse and nourish the body with **diet**, juicing, fasting, and exercise; quiet and focus the mind with journaling and meditation; and renew and awaken the spirit with study, prayer and celebration.

Cleansing and Nourishing Your Body:

Your body is self-healing. When given the proper tools to work with, it can restore itself to its natural balance.

Practiced for many centuries around the world, detoxification is the process of cleansing the body to promote healing and longevity. To help your body cleanse and restore itself, OHI provides:

- **Wheatgrass juice** to cleanse cells and purify blood
- **Enemas** and **wheatgrass implants** to cleanse the colon
- **Gentle exercise** to cleanse the lymphatic system

OHI contracts with qualified professionals to make optional services available to you. These services supplement the core OHI holistic healing program:

- **Massages and spa treatments** to remove congestion and release tension
- **Colon hydrotherapy** to eliminate toxins
- **Chiropractic** care to reduce structural or nerve pain

Contact information:

Optimum Health Institute of San Diego

6970 Central Avenue
Lemon Grove, CA 91945

Call to make a reservation

(800) 993-4325
(619) 464-3346

Optimum Health Institute of Austin

265 Cedar Lane
Cedar Creek, TX 78612

Call to make a reservation

(800) 993-4325
(512) 303-4817

Website: http://www.optimumhealth.org

Chapter 12

Herbal Recipes used for Centuries to Kill Cancer cells

*"**Inaction** breeds **doubt** and **fear**. **Action** breeds **confidence** and **courage**. If you want **to conquer fear**, do **not** sit home and think about it. **Go out and get busy.**"*

Dale Carnegie

Herbal treatments are documented as the oldest type of approach to cancer and have been **used with success for thousands of years by indigenous people all around the world.**

In recent years, modern science has proven that many herbs do, in fact, have **cancer-fighting properties**. They have been shown to support the body's **immune system**, improve **blood circulation**, strengthen the functioning of major organs, and enhance the efficient **elimination of toxins**, among other things. **They can act very much like a potent drug as well.** For instance, some herbs have direct **cytotoxic effects** on the cancer cells themselves, while not harming other cells of the body. Other herbs have been shown to inhibit a tumor's ability to produce **new blood vessels** to feed itself, thereby strangling the tumor's system of nourishment. And still other herbs have **anti-microbial properties**. Thus, herbs are often referred to as "nature's medicine" and the **Hoxsey therapy for cancer is a wonderful example of this that I will now share with you.**

The Hoxsey Therapy

The Hoxsey therapy was the first widely used alternative non-toxic treatment for cancer in the modern United States. Still obtainable today, it is a treatment that consists of an herbal topical salve, an herbal topical powder, and an herbal internal tonic. Though many people have never heard of it, this treatment approach was very successful and was actually used by tens of thousands of Americans in the early to mid-1900s. Around 1953, at the height of the Hoxsey therapy, the main Hoxsey clinic in Dallas, Texas had 12,000 patients and was the largest private cancer center in the world. There were also subsidiary clinics in 17 other states.

History

Harry Hoxsey, an American who lived from 1901 to 1974, was the person responsible for the widespread use of the Hoxsey therapy for cancer. The herbal remedy had been passed down to Harry by his great-grandfather, John Hoxsey. It was John Hoxsey, a horse breeder in Illinois, who developed the herbal remedy. In 1840 Harry's great-grandfather John had a stallion that was expected to die as a result of having developed a cancerous lesion on its leg. This horse had been one of John's favorites, so when the horse had to be put out to pasture, he kept an eye on it. He noticed that the horse exhibited atypical behavior by grazing primarily on one clump of shrubs and flowering plants. He also noticed that the horse's cancer completely healed after a number of months and the stallion made a full recovery.

Curious about his horse's amazing return to health, John picked samples from the plants on which the stallion had been grazing. Through experimentation, he developed an herbal tonic, salve, and powder from them. Some think John Hoxsey may have also gotten input from some of the local Native Americans about the use of these plants. He then started using these remedies to treat other horses suffering from external cancers or other types of lesions. John's herbal mixture proved to be quite successful, and word spread quickly until horse breeders were bringing their horses to him from as far away as Indiana and Kentucky.

John Hoxsey's herbal mixtures were eventually passed down to Harry's father, a veterinarian. Harry's father used the herbal remedies to treat animals with cancer and other conditions. But he started to quietly use the herbal treatments to help humans with cancer as well.

When Harry was eight years old, he began assisting his father in administering these treatments to some of the local people. These were generally people who had no other hope for recovery, and the Hoxsey remedies were having success. Just before his father's death, Harry, the youngest in a family of 12 children, was entrusted with the secrets of how to prepare the remedies and was given the responsibility to carry on the family's healing tradition.

The Hoxsey therapy was mostly known for its success with external tumors on the surface of the body. People with external cancers were treated with an herbal paste applied directly onto the tumor and given a liquid herbal tonic to drink as well. People with **internal cancer** that showed no external signs were just given the Hoxsey's tonic. Certain dietary changes were also recommended to patients in general, along with a few nutritional supplements.

The Hoxsey Tonic ingredients:

RED CLOVER BLOSSOM
LICORICE ROOT
BUCKTHORN BARK
BURDOCK ROOT
STILLINGIA ROOT
POKE ROOT
BARBERRY ROOT
OREGON GRAPE ROOT
CASCARA SAGRADA BARK
PRICKLY ASH BARK
WILD INDIGO ROOT
SEA KELP
POTASSIUM IODIDE

Though it was not proven at the time, botanists have since found all of the herbs in the Hoxsey tonic to have various anti-cancer properties. And the external salve contains bloodroot, which has been used by Native Americans to treat cancer for centuries.

Ranch wife Della Mae Nelson had uterine cancer that had been extensively treated with twenty units of X-ray and thirty-six hours of radium. She was so badly burned from the radiation that she couldn't even pull a sheet over her body for a year after. Wasted to eighty-six pounds, she was bleeding internally, so severely impaired that she had to learn to walk all over again. Then the cancer recurred.

When Della Mae's cancer recurred, her conventional doctors told the family there was nothing more they could do for her. Against her daughter's wishes, Della Mae then sought treatment at the Hoxsey clinic in Dallas. She, too, completely recovered from her cancer as a result of the Hoxsey therapy. (Della Mae Nelson died about 50 years later, in 1997, at the age of ninety-nine. She had outlived most of the conventional doctors and nurses that had treated her).

All of the Hoxsey clinics admitted and treated any cancer patient who came to them, even *those that could not pay.* Ausubel's book documents numerous times when Hoxsey exhibited generosity to his patients above and beyond the call of duty, including fully treating people who had used up their last dime on bus fare to get to the clinic. Many times Hoxsey then drove them to a local place where they could stay. In reality, Hoxsey was following the advice his father had given him when he handed the responsibility of the family remedies over. His father said:

"Now you have the power to heal the sick and save lives. What I've managed to do in a tiny part of this state, you can do all over the country, all over the world. I've cured hundreds of people. You can cure thousands, tens of thousands.

But it's not only a gift, son; it's a trust and a great responsibility. Abe Lincoln once said God must have loved the common people because he made so many of them. We're common, ordinary people. You must never refuse to treat anybody because he can't pay. Promise me that!"

In 1954, an independent group of 10 doctors from various parts of the United States made a point of investigating Hoxsey's clinic in Dallas. After the two-day inspection, which included examining hundreds of case histories and talking to patients and ex-patients, this independent group of physicians made a stunning public conclusion. **They reported that the Hoxsey clinic is successfully treating pathologically proven cases of cancer, both internal and external, without the use of surgery, radium or x-ray.**

Accepting the standard yardstick of cases that have remained symptom- free in excess of five to six years after treatment, established by medical authorities, we have seen sufficient cases to warrant such a conclusion. Some of those presented before us have been free of symptoms as long as twenty-four years, and the physical evidence indicates that they are all enjoying exceptional health at this time.

Doctors' CONCLUSION:

We as a Committee feel that the Hoxsey treatment is superior to such conventional methods of treatment as x-ray, radium, and surgery.

Current Hoxsey Therapy

The Bio-Medical Center in Tijuana continues to operate and administer the Hoxsey therapy. Information below indicates how to contact this treatment center.

Contact information:

BIOMEDICAL CENTER

Location: 3170 General Ferreira Col. Juarez - Tijuana, Baja California - 22150 MEXICO

Mailing address: PO box 433654 - San Isidro, CA 92143 - 3654

Telephone: (011-52664) 684-90-11 - Fax: (011-52664) 684-97-44

In addition to the Hoxsey treatment, comprised of a liquid elixir containing a mixture of herbs and several topical salves, the clinic may also use other supplements, diet, nutrition, and chelation therapy. They treat most types of malignancies, but it is said to be especially effective with skin cancer (including melanoma), breast cancer, and has been successful with some recurrent cancers and even with patients who've had radiation and/or chemotherapy.

I also think you will be interested to read about another powerful herbal recipe:

Essiac Tea

*"Put **LOVE** first. Entertain thoughts that give life. And when a thought or resentment, or hurt, or fear comes your way, have another thought that is more powerful – a thought that is **LOVE**"*

Mary Morrissey

Essiac Tea is a long proven method of curing cancer. It dates back to the 1920s and before.

What is the history of the discovery and use of Essiac and Flor Essence as complementary or alternative treatments for cancer?

Essiac was created by a Canadian nurse called Renee Caisse. She named the remedy after herself - Essiac is her surname spelled backwards. Other names for Essiac include 'Flor essence' and 'tea of life'. Renee Caisse first began to promote Essiac as a cancer treatment in the 1920s. Today, Essiac and Flor Essence may be sold as herbal supplements as long as they do not claim to treat or cure cancer.

- In 1922, a breast cancer patient gave the Essiac formula to the nurse and said it had cured her disease. The patient said the formula came from an Ontario Ojibwa Native American medicine man.

- In 1934, the nurse opened a cancer clinic in Ontario and gave Essiac to patients free of charge. In 1938, the Royal Cancer Commission of Canada visited the clinic but found little evidence that Essiac was effective. The nurse closed the clinic in 1942 but continued to give Essiac to patients until the late 1970s.

- Between 1959 and the late 1970s, the nurse worked with an American doctor to study Essiac in the laboratory and in people and to promote its use. They also created the formula now called Flor Essence. The results of their studies were not reported in any peer-reviewed scientific journals. Most scientific journals have experts who review research reports before they are published, to make sure that the evidence and conclusions are sound. Studies published in peer-reviewed scientific journals are considered to be better evidence.

In the 1980s, companies making Essiac-like products began to sell the mixtures as health tonics. Because these companies did not make claims that it would treat or cure certain diseases, Essiac did not come under laws that regulate it as a drug.

While the basic components of Essiac are well known, the exact proportions of the herbs in Essiac are the matter of much speculation. The cancer patient should be far more concerned with the quality of the herbs, and the quality of the processing, than with the exact formula. Some brands have 4, 6 or 8 herbs (e.g. Flor-Essence has 8 herbs). The extra herbs won't hurt, and may be of some help. But again, the quality of the herbs, and the quality of the processing, is the most important issue.

It should be mentioned that it is the **Sheep Sorrel** that is the **main cancer-killing herb** in Essiac. Sheep Sorrel has been known about for over a hundred years as a **cancer-fighting herb**.

© Natalie Mitchell

The Four Main Essiac Tea Ingredients:

Burdock Root

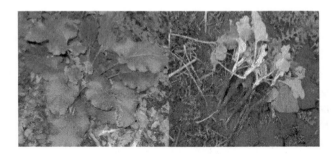

Burdock root has been known to be an effective blood purifier for centuries now. Its seeds contain oil that is eliminated through sweating; taking poisons and toxins with it and it also helps heal some skin problems. Burdock root also contains niacin, which is known for ridding the body of toxins, like those absorbed through radiation. Burdock root also is been known to dissolve kidney stones, as well as provide support for the bladder and liver. Minerals such as iron are abundant in this root. Studies have also shown that burdock can help shrink tumors or prevent it from growing. This property of Burdock root that prevents mutations is called the "B factor". The Japanese, who also use Burdock root in medicine, discovered this. The World Health Organization has also reported that Burdock is a potential treatment for HIV because it appears to be active against the virus. The extract form of Burdock root reportedly demonstrated strong anti-cancer activity against leukemia. Burdock is also used in another herbal cancer treatment you read about above which is **Hoxsey cancer treatment**. Check out this page to read more about burdock root benefits.

Sheep Sorrel

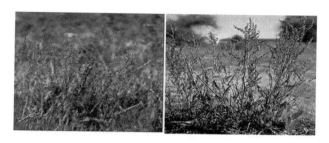

Sheep sorrel, when taken in different forms, yields different results. As a cool drink, it may lower your temperature if you have a fever. When taken as a tea, it is good for stomach pains and diarrhea. It could also be gargled, to alleviate sore throats. Its astringent properties also have been known to stop internal or external bleeding although it is recommended that you seek medical attention immediately instead of self-medicating with sheep sorrel.

Since sheep sorrel is high in antioxidants, it helps to protect cells from damage due to normal cell metabolism and/or destruction. Aside from having anti-tumor properties, it also appears to be an antiseptic and antibacterial. Some studies show strong evidence that this shrinks tumors in humans, while the other uses were mostly tested on mice. People suffering from arthritis can also find use for this as it has anti-inflammatory properties as well. Like fruits and vegetables, sheep sorrel contains many vitamins and minerals that could alleviate pains due to stress, fatigue, and other aches.

Its uses are related to the circulatory system, indicating that those who are suffering imbalances of this nature can benefit from this herb. Some less popular theories even claim that it has anti-angiogenesis properties. That basically means this herb may have the power to cut off the main energy source of tumors. This avenue of treatment is currently being studied as another way to cure cancer.

Slippery Elm Bark

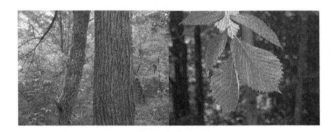

Before it was discovered for its medicinal purposes, this tree was made into houses, canoes, baskets and more. Soldiers relied on this as their food source to help them survive when lost at war.

The inner bark of this tree is mostly used for its soothing effects. In fact, it is considered safe enough for infants as well as pregnant women and the elderly. The soothing effects stem from its high mucilage content. Mucilage serves to strengthen and heal tissues. Before a tissue heals, it has to be soothed and stabilized from any prior irritation. Organs of the body that benefit most from this are the lungs, intestines and urinary tracts. It is a go-to food when one can barely ingest anything and is even as nutritious as oats. It's an excellent source of calcium, which is good for the nervous system and emotional wellbeing. A constituent called tannins makes this herb an astringent as well. When made into a paste, it can sooth wounds, burns, boils and other inflamed or painful surfaces. It is also reportedly used for drawing out the poison from a bullet wound.

Turkey Rhubarb Root

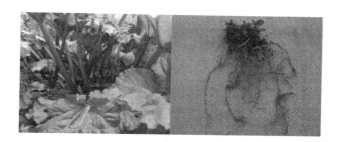

The name Turkey Rhubarb came to be from its early days as an export of China. This was mainly used for two cases: diarrhea and constipation. Smaller doses would help cease the sometimes-involuntary expulsion of waste, as larger doses were administered to help alleviate constipation.

It is a popular ingredient in many Chinese medicinal recipes. It also reportedly improves symptoms of kidney failure. It is an anti-tumor, anti-inflammatory, anti-bacterial and is more palatable than its counterpart, garden rhubarb root.

Turkish rhubarb is one of the most-discussed Essiac tea ingredients.

Essiac Tea Benefits: Primary Actions

Essiac tea's primary actions are to remove heavy metals, detoxify the body, restore energy levels, and rebuild the immune system. After this occurs, the body is restored to a level to where it is able to better defeat an illness or disease state *using its own resources.*

Everyone comes in contact with viruses and bacteria all the time, and everyone is susceptible to developing health problems. *People only get sick because their body's immune system FAILS to fight off the illness or infection.* Therefore if the immune system is boosted, many illnesses and diseases can be eradicated WITH NO DRUGS. Essiac tea benefits the immune system more than any other substance we know of.

Here are some ESSIAC TEA benefits that have been reported and observed in research performed by Rene Caisse and Dr. Charles Brusch at the Brusch Medical Research Center.

Essiac Tea...

1. Prevents the buildup of excess fatty deposits in artery walls, heart, kidney and liver.

2. Regulates cholesterol levels by transforming sugar and fat into energy.

3. Destroys parasites in the digestive system and throughout the body.

4. Counteracts the effects of aluminum, lead and mercury poisoning.

5. Strengthens and improves the functioning of muscles, organs and tissues.

6. Makes bones, joints, ligaments, lungs, and membranes strong and flexible, and therefore less vulnerable to stress or stress injuries.

7. Nourishes and stimulates the brain and nervous system.

8. Promotes the absorption of fluids in the tissues.

9. Removes toxic accumulations in the fat, lymph, bone marrow, bladder, and alimentary canals.

10. Neutralizes acids, absorbs toxins in the bowel, and eliminates both.

11. Clears the respiratory channels by dissolving and expelling mucus.

12. Relieves the liver of its burden of detoxification by converting fatty toxins into water-soluble substances that can then be easily eliminated through the kidneys.

13. Assists the liver to produce lecithin, which forms part of the myelin sheath, a white fatty material that encloses nerve fibers.

14. Reduces, perhaps eliminates, heavy metal deposits in tissues (especially those surrounding the joints) to reduce inflammation and stiffness.

15. Improves the functions of the pancreas and spleen by increasing the effectiveness of insulin.

16. Purifies the blood.

17. Increases red cell production, and keeps them from rupturing.

18. Increases the body's ability to utilize oxygen by raising the oxygen level in the tissue cells.

19. Maintains the balance between potassium and sodium within the body so that the fluid inside and outside each cell is regulated; in this way, cells are nourished with nutrients and are also cleansed properly.

20. Converts calcium and potassium oxalates into a harmless form by making them solvent in the urine. Regulates the amount of oxalic acid delivered to the kidneys, thus reducing the risk of stone formation in the gall bladder, kidneys, or urinary tract.

21. Protects against toxins entering the brain.

22. Protects the body against radiation and X-rays.

23. Relieves pain.

24. Speeds up wound healing by regenerating the damaged area.

25. Increases the production of antibodies like lymphocytes and T-cells in the thymus gland, which is the defender of our immune system.

26. Protects the cells against free radicals.

27. Increases the appetite for healthful foods.

28. Decreases sugar cravings due to better blood sugar control.

29. Increases energy available.

30. Boosts mood and leads to an improved sense of well being.

Testimonials from cancer patients who achieved complete remission or considerable improvement using **Essiac** are obtainable from Elaine Alexander. These remarkable letters document cases of the last fifteen years and encompass **many types of cancer, including pancreatic, breast, and ovarian cancer; cancers of the esophagus, bile ducts, bladder, and bones; and lymphoma and metastatic melanoma.**

Muriel Peters of Creston, British Columbia, one of the people who wrote to Elaine Alexander to describe her experience with Essiac, was diagnosed in 1981 with a malignant tumor the size of an orange on her coccyx, the triangular bone at the base of the spine. She underwent surgery a week later. The surgeons told her, "We got it all," but according to Muriel, "By the time they had found the tumor, it had begun to flare up the spine among the nerve endings, so they could not cut there." She had twenty-nine radiation treatments following the surgery. In September 1982, sensing numbness in her lower abdominal area, she went to the Cancer Clinic in Vancouver and was told by a head surgeon that the tumor had spread to her spine and was inoperable, and nothing more could be done.

When her brother-in-law mentioned a man with cancer who had been given three months to live but was cured "somewhere down South," Muriel Peters followed up the lead. One month later, she visited the Bio-Medical Center in Tijuana, Mexico, and began the Hoxsey herbal therapy. Within three months, sensation returned to her lower abdomen, but this was followed by "three months of excruciating pain which no pills could relieve." She then began taking Essiac in liquid form, which she obtained from the Resperin Corporation through her doctor. After twelve days, the pain subsided. "From then on I was on my way up."

For the next year and a half, Muriel took Essiac daily. She also remained on the Hoxsey regimen, which consisted of an herbal tonic, vitamin supplements, and a special diet stressing fresh vegetables, greens, and fruits. "I felt the two complemented each other," Muriel explains. "Without the diet and the vitamins, I really doubt if either of the tonics would have been quite enough. The body has to rebuild what the cancer has broken down; therefore healthy foods are needed by the body to reconstruct itself."

About a year after she started her dual program, Muriel returned for tests to the Vancouver Cancer Clinic. Incredulous, the attending doctor told her, "For reasons unknown there have been notable changes in your body."

"When the doctor left the room," recalls Muriel, "the attending nurse asked me what I was doing to bring about these changes, and I only said, 'I'm on a diet and vitamins.' The nurse asked, 'On your own?' I replied, 'No, by doctors directing.' She then said, 'Well, as long as you're not going to Mexican quacks, as many are doing.'"

A complete medical checkup in September 1989 found Muriel Peters cancer-free and in excellent health. At sixty-eight, she reported, "I'm the healthiest person in British Columbia. I love life and living.... I have learned what life is all about." X-rays and blood tests in January 1991 confirmed her to be in complete remission, nine years after she was diagnosed with inoperable, **"hopeless" cancer.**

Chapter 13

The Connection between Your Mind, Body and Emotions

*"The **Mind** in itself and in its own place can make a hell out of **Heaven** or a **Heaven** out of hell"*

John Milton

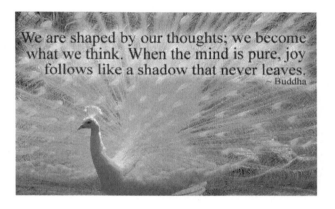

We are shaped by our thoughts; we become what we think. When the mind is pure, joy follows like a shadow that never leaves.
~ Buddha

Legendary psychologist and Holocaust-survivor Viktor Frankl once wrote, "Everything can be taken from a person but one thing: the last of human freedoms - to choose one's attitudes in any given set of circumstances, **to choose one's own way**." Frankl was right. **Attitude is a personal choice for all of us**. You could be faced with a thousand problems, many or most over which you have absolutely no control. However, there is always one thing you are in complete and absolute control of and that is your **own attitude** and therefore your actions!

Attitude is the composite of **your thoughts, feelings, emotions** and **actions**. Your **conscious mind** controls **feelings** and ultimately dictates whether your feelings will be **positive** or **negative** by your **choice of thoughts**, then your body displays those choices through **action** and **behavior.**

Attitude is actually a **creative cycle** that begins with your **choice of thoughts**. You **do** choose your thoughts and that choice is where your attitude originates. As you internalize ideas or become emotionally involved with your thoughts, you create the second stage in forming an attitude; you move your entire being - mind and body - into a new "vibration." Your conscious awareness of this vibration is referred to as "feelings". Your feelings are then expressed in actions or behaviors that produce the various results in your life.

Positive results are always the effect of a **positive attitude**.

Attitude and results are inseparable.

Simply stated, if you think in **negative terms**, you will get **negative results**; if you think in **positive terms** you will achieve **positive results**. Ralph Waldo Emerson reiterated that same point when he said, **"A person is what they think about all day long."** The results you achieve in life are nothing more than an expression of your **thoughts, feelings**, and **actions**.

Winning and **losing** are opposite sides of the same coin -

and that coin *is attitude.* There are many things wrong in this world; unfortunately that is all some people are able to see. Those who view the world in this light are often unhappy and somewhat cynical. Usually, their life is one of lack and limitation and it almost appears as if they move from one bad experience to another. I know people who are like this and I'm certain you do as well. It would appear as if they were born with a streak of bad luck and it has followed them around their whole life. These individuals are quick to **blame circumstances** or other **people** for their problems, rather than accepting **responsibility** for their life and their **attitude**.

Conversely, there are others who are forever winning and living the good life. They are the real movers and shakers who make things happen. They seem to go from one major accomplishment to another. They're in control of their life; they know where they are going and **know they will get there**. They are the **real winners** in life and their wins are a matter of their **choice**.

Let's speaks about worries and stress. Something I would like you to know is that **stress affects blood flow** within the body. Not everybody knows about this connection, otherwise people would pay more attention to their reactions and attitude. When the body becomes stressed, it channels more blood to the muscles of the arms and legs, causing less blood to go to the stomach. As a result, food is more slowly digested and instead remains in the stomach for longer periods of time. **Undigested food** is one of the primary causes of **acid** reflux as the food pushes up against the top of the stomach, opening a valve called the lower esophageal sphincter. When undigested food causes this sphincter to open, this allows acid to reflux back up from the stomach into the esophagus. This is one way in which increased stress can cause acid reflux.

We saw in earlier chapters how dangerous an acidic body environment is for us. Imagine how bad it is for the body if people eat acidic food on top of being stressed. Even if do everything else do make your body more alkaline and at the same time you are stressed and worried, the body will still produce dangerous acidity. If you stop and just think about your inner feelings, emotions, attitude to life you realize that it is only **you** who decides how to react to certain circumstances and what an attitude towards life to have. You are a Master of your own choice of emotions, thought, feelings and actions!

Think about this…

During the day average person have approximately sixty thousands thoughts, and guess what: 85% of them exactly the same ones they had the day before and even worse that a lot of them are negative.

You may have heard or read the expression in the Bible "Drink water from your own well". You saw above the percentage of water our body and brain contains. So what is the quality of our water are when we allow ourselves to think negative thoughts and emotions? No wonder why many of us feel constantly exhausted.

Worry drains us of our natural vitality and energy. If you have a bicycle and its tires are fully inflated it will take you to your destination, when a tire has a leak it will deflate eventually and interrupt the journey. The same analogy can be applied with worry; it only causes your precious mental energy and potential to leak away, just like air leaking out of a tire.

Again it is in your own hands to stop worrying and invest your precious energy to get healthier with the knowledge your mind is equipped now. You can enjoy inner peace that you are doing everything to give your blood cells the highest opportunity to do the best for you.

One of the good techniques for ridding the mind of worry and other negative, life-draining influences is when any negative thought comes to your mind as they do so to all of us, to say "thank you" to that one and to then replace it with a positive thought. It is a very simple technique known for centuries as our mind can only hold one thought at any one time. Using this technique, anyone can easily create a positive, creative mind set within a short period of time. It is one or the other: your mind controls you or you control your mind. You are the Master of your thoughts and only you can decide which one you allow to enter your precious Mind!

In reality, the quality of your thinking determines the quality of your life. A strong, disciplined mind, which anyone can cultivate through daily practice, leads to powerful actions and as a result positive and desirable change!

We must be grateful and appreciative for everything we have and how often we forget to express that thought. The more we are thankful to God and people surrounding us for all we have and experienced on this beautiful planet the more positive change we will attract to our life.

Your positive mind will be a huge help for your beloved blood cells as they will be able to perform in completely different mode and you will see the transformation.

When you wake up in the morning ask yourself a question: "How am I going to enjoy myself today?" Think about it and include something in your day that you would love to do and do it for.

Dorothea Brand once said, *"Act as if it were impossible to fail,"* and I challenge you to do so. By simply becoming aware that you can choose what to nourish your body with, concentrating on positive thoughts, emotions, being grateful and as a result acting in this focused way each and every day, you will achieve your goal. You have to decide right now what you are going to do with your body, as you are its Master, and with your thoughts and emotions - and take an action.

You have the power to choose what you give your body to work with, no matter what your circumstances are. That positive personal choice will allow your blood cells to do the best work for your entire body and you can be healthier and more energetic! You don't have to be a prisoner of your past instead you can become an Architect of your present and future!

God Bless You!

*"Yesterday is a **history**, tomorrow is a **mystery**, **today is a gift of God**, which is why we call it the present."*

Bill Keane

References:

Airola, Ph.D., Paavo, How to Get Well, Health Plus, Sherwood, Oregon, 1993.

Altschul, Aaron M. Proteins, Their Chemistry and Politics, Basic Books, New York, 1965.

Barefoot, Robert R. And Carl J. Reich, M.D., The Calcium Factor: The Scientific Secret of Health and Youth, Gilliland Printing Inc., Arkansas City, Kansas, 1996.

Binzel, M.D., Philip E., Alive and Well - One Doctor's Experience with Nutrition in the Treatment of Cancer Patients, American Media. Westlake Village, CA, 1994. "In my attempts to use nutritional therapy, which includes the use of Laetrile, in the treatment of cancer, I have often been confronted by the Food and Drug Administration and by the State Medical Board. I have fought and, through the grace of God, I have won."

Budwig, Dr. Johanna, Flax Oil As a True Aid Against Arthritis, Heart Infarction, Cancer and Other Diseases, Apple Publishing Company Ltd., Vancouver, 1996.

Day, Phillip, Cancer - Why We're Still Dying To Know The Truth, Credence Publications, PO Box 3, Tonbridge, Kent TN12 9ZY, United Kingdom.

Diamond, M.D., W. John, W. Lee Cowden, M.D. with Burton Goldberg, An Alternative Medicine Definitive Guide to Cancer, Future Medicine Publishing, Inc., Tiburon, California, 1997.

Erasmus, Ph.D., Udo, Fats that Heal, Fats that Kill, Alive Books, 1993.

Fife, N.D., Bruce, The Coconut Oil Miracle, Avery, New York, 2004.

Fuhrman, M.D., Joel, Eat To Live: The Revolutionary Formula for Fast and Sustained Weight Loss, Little Brown, 2003.

Gerson, M.D., Max, A Cancer Therapy - Results of Fifty Cases and The Cure of Advanced Cancer by Diet Therapy - A Summary of 30 Years of Clinical Experimentation, Gerson Institute, Binita, California, 1990.

Griffin, G. Edward, World Without Cancer, American Media, Westlake Village, California, 1997. Both the book and video can be purchased directly from the author.

Jochems, Ruth, Dr. Moerman's Anti-Cancer Diet, Avery Publishing Group Inc., Garden City Park, New York, 1990. In Holland the vegetarian diet promoted by Dr. Moerman has been recognized by the government as a legitimate treatment for cancer. Results indicate that Dr. Moerman's diet is more effective than standard cancer treatments.

Kelley, Dr. William Donald, Cancer: Curing the Incurable Without Surgery, Chemotherapy, or Radiation, 2001. Newly revised and updated information from Dr. Kelley.

Kendall, Roger V., Building Wellness with DMG - How a breakthrough nutrient gives cancer, autism & cardiovascular patients a second chance at health, Freedom Press, 2003.

Lappe, Frances Moore, Diet for a Small Planet, Ballantine Books, New York, 1992. This book explains the principle of protein complementarity that is the basis of the vegetarian diet. By combining a grain and a legume you produce a protein that is as good as animal protein. Examples include: rice and lentils (rice and dahl - India), corn and beans (Mexico), chick peas and wheat (falafel sandwich - Middle East). This famous bread recipe takes full advantage of protein complementarity: "Take wheat and barley, beans and lentils, millet and spelt; put them in a storage jar and use them to make bread for yourself." - Ezekiel 4:9. A high protein plant diet provides twice the vitamins and minerals of a meat diet, and vastly more fiber, phyto-nutrients, and other required nutrients.

McDaniel, T.C., Disease Reprieve, Xlibris Corporation, 1999. Understanding zeta potential and human health.

McTaggart, Lynne, What Doctors Don't Tell You, First Avon Books, New York, 1998.

Montignac, Michel, Eat Yourself Slim, Alex & Lucas Publishing, 2004.

Pierce, N.D., Carson E., What I Would Do If I Had Cancer Again, 1996.

Robbins, John, Reclaiming Our Health, H J Kramer Inc., Tiburon, California, 1998.

Sharma, M.D., Hari, Freedom from Disease, Veda Publishing, Toronto, Ontario, 1993.

Sharma, M.D., Hari, et al, The Answer To Cancer Is Never Giving It A Chance to Start, Select Books, New York, 2002.

Taylor, Ross, with forward by Olivia Newton-John, Living Simply With Cancer, Cancer Support Association, Perth, Western Australia, 1998.

Whang, Sang, Reverse Aging, Siloam Enterprise, Inc., Englewood Cliffs, NJ, 1994.

Young, M.D., Robert O., The pH Miracle: Balance Your Diet; Reclaim Your Health, Wellness Central, 2003. See also Dr. Young's website.

Clinical Oncology for Medical Students and Physicians, op. cit, pp.32, 34

Spontaneous Regression of Cancer: "The Metabolic Triumph of the Host!", op. cit.,pp. 136, 137.

Manner, HW, Michaelson, TL, and DiSanti, SJ. "Enzymatic Analysis of Normal and Malignant Tissues." Presented at the Illinois State Academy of Science, April 1978. Also, Manner, HW, Michaelson, TL, and DiSanti, SJ, "Amygdalin, Vitamin A and Enzymes Induced Regression of Murine Mammary Adenocarcinomas", Journal of Manipulative and Physiological Therapeutics, Vol 1, No. 4, December 1978. 200 East Roosevelt Road, Lombard, IL 60148 USA

Vitamin B15 (Pangamic Acid); Properties, Functions, and Use. (Moscow: Science Publishing House, 1965), translated and reprinted by McNaughton Foundation, Sausalito, Calif.

Catalona, et al. Medical World News, 6/23/72, pg 82M California cancer Advisory council, 1963, pg 10 Weilerstein, R. W., ACS Volunteer, 19, #1, 1973

Burger, Hospital Practice, July, 1973, 55-62

Currie & Bagshawe, Lancet, 1, (7492), 708, 1967

Abercrombie, Ca. Res. 22, 525, 1962

Cormack, Ca. Res. 30, (5), 1459, 1970

Catalona, et al. Medical World News, 6/23/72, pg 82M

Jose, Nut. Today, March, 1973, pgs 4-9

Burk & Winzler, VITAMINS AND HORMONES, vol. II, 1944

Adcock et al, Science, 181, 8/31/73, 845-47

Dr. Dean Burk formerly chief of cytochemistry, The National cancer institute, and

Dr. John Yiamouyiannis, Science Director of The National Health Federation, Formerly an editor of chemical Abstracts.
Fairley, Brit. Med. J. 2,1969, 467-473
Burk, McNaughton, Von Ardenne, PanMinerva Med. 13, #12, Dec. 1971
Lea, et al, ca. Res. 35, 2321 -2326, Sept. 1975
The McNaughton Foundation, I.N.D. 6734, April 6, 1970
Nieper, Krebsgeschehen, 4,1972
J.A.M.A. 225, 4, July, 1973, pg 424
Shamberger et al, Proc. Nat, Acad. Sci. May, 1973
Shute & Shute, ALPHA TOCOPHEROL IN CARDIOVASCULAR DISEASE, Ryerson Press, Toronto, Canada, 1954
Ransberger, 10th Int. Cancer Congress, 1970
Wolf & Ransberger, ENZYME THERAPY, Vantage Pr. 1972
Summa; Dipl. Ing. (Chem) Landstuhl, 1972
Reitnauer, Arzneim. Forsch. 22, 1347-61, 1972
Folkman, Ann. Surg. 175, (3). 409-1 6, 1972
Penn, 7th Annual Cancer Conf. 1973
The MEDICAL LETTER, vol. 15, #3 (issue #367) 2/2/73
Kreuger, ADVANCES IN PHARM. & CHEMOTHERAPY, vol x, 1973
Annals New York Academy of Science: 164, 2, 1969
Sorbo, Acta Chem. Scand. 5, 1951, (724-34); 1953 (1129-1136); 1953 (1137-1145)

Clemedson et al, Acta Physiol. Scand. 32, 1954, 245
Engel, Med. Klink. 20, 1790, 1930
DeFermo, Arch. Ital. de Chir. 33: 801, 1933
Saphir,~Endocrinol. 18, 191, 1934
Velasquez & Engel, Endocrinol. 27, 523, 1940
Li, Med. Clin N. Am. 45, 661 -666, May, 1961
Roffo, Bol. Inst. de Med. 21, 41 9-586, 1944
Friedman, Ann. N.Y. Acad. Sci. 80-1 61, 1959 (and refs)
Krebs & Gurchot, Science, 104, 302, 1946
Braunstein, et al, Annals Int. Med. 78:39-45, 1973
Naughton et al, Ca. Res. 35, 1887-1 890, July, 1975
Wide & Gemzell, Acta Endocrinol. 35-261, 1960
Navarro, 9th International Cancer Congress, Toyko, Oct. 1966 reported in HEALTH AND LIGHT, by John Ott, D.Sc., Devin Adair, 1973
Nieper, Agressologie 12, 6,1971, 401-8
Livingston, CANCER: A NEW BREAKTHROUGH, Nash Publishing, Los Angeles, 1972
Benno C. Schmidt, chairman of the Memorial Sloan-Kettering Cancer Center, New York City, chairman of The President's Cancer Panel; address to the A.C.S., California Division, Oct. 12, 1973 (Los Angeles Times)
Yudkin, SWEET AND DANGEROUS, Bantam Books, 1972
Seminars on Healing, The Academy of Parapsychology and Medicine, June 1973

Torrance & Schnabel, Ann. Intern. Med. 6, 732, 1932
Leivy & Schnabel, Am. I. Med. Sd. 183, 381, 1932
Gillette, et al, I. Clin. Invest. 51, 36a, 1972
Gillette, et al, New Eng. J. Med. 290, 654, 1974

Cerami & Manning, Prac. Natl. Acad. Sci. 68, 1180, 1971
Gillette et al, ibid, 68, 2791, 1971
Cerami, et al, Fed. Proc. 32, 1668, 1973
Manning, et al, Adv. Exp. Med. Biol. 28, 253, 1972
Houston, Am. Laboratory, 7, #10, October, 1975 (and editorial)
DeLange & Ermans, Am. I. Clin. Nut. 24, 1354, 1971
Barnes, Broda, M.D., HEART ATTACK RARENESS IN THYROID-TREATED PA
TIENTS, C.C. Thomas, 1972
Barnes and Galton, HYPOTHYROIDISM, THE UNSUSPECTED ILLNESS,
Thomas Y. Crowell, N.Y., Feb. 1976
Smith, J. C. Medical Counterpoint, Nov. 1973
Oberleas, Intntl. Trace Elements Symp. Modern Med., Sept. 16, 1974
New Scientist, 5/2/74
Korant, B.D., Nature, 4/12/74
Klenner, FR., I. So. Med. & Surg. 111, 209, 1949
Stacpoole, P.W., Med. Hyp., March-April, 1975
C.A. Dombradi and S. Foldeak, "Screening Report on the Antitumor Activity of
Purified Arctium Lappa Extracts," Tumori, vol. 52, 1966, p. 173, cited in Patricia
Spain Ward, "History of Hoxsey Treatment," contract report for the U.S. Congress,
Office of Technology Assessment, May 1988.
Kazuyoshi Morita, Tsuneo Kada, and Mitsuo Namiki, "A Desmutagenic Factor
Isolated From Burdock (Arctium Lappa Linne)," Mutation Research, vol. 129,
1984, pp. 25-31, cited in Patricia Spain Ward, "History of Hoxsey Treatment,"
contract report for the U.S. Congress, Office of Technology Assessment, May
1988.

Sheila Snow Fraser and Carroll Allen, "Could Essiac Halt Cancer?" Homemaker's,
June-July August 1977, p. 19.
"Essiac as an Aid in Surgery," Bracebridge Examiner, 13 March 1991.
Gary L. Glum, Calling of an Angel (Los Angeles: Silent Walker Publishing, 1988),
p. i. "Essiac Added 18 Years to Her Mother's Life," Bracebridge Examiner, 6
February 1991. 7. "Cancer Commission Was Nothing But a Farce," Bracebridge
Examiner, 9 January 1991. 8. Glum, op. cit., p. 136.9. Ibid.

S. J. Haught. Censured for Curing Cancer: The American Experience of Dr. Max
Gerson. San Diego: The Gerson Institute, 1991.
Tanya Harter Pierce M.A., MFCC, "Outsmart your cancer" 2004.
Richard Walters. Options: The Alternative Cancer Therapy Book. New York: Avery
Penguin Putnam, 1993.

James P. Carter, M.D. Racketeering in Medicine: The Suppression of Alter-
natives. Hampton Roads, 1993.
Ross Pelton and Lee Overholser. Alternatives in Cancer Therapy. New York:
Simon and Schuster, 1994.
Nicholas A Graham, Martik Tahmasian, Bitika Kohli, Evangelia Komisopoulou,
Maggie Zhu, Igor Vivanco, Michael A Teitell, Hong Wu, Antoni Ribas, Roger S Lo,
Ingo K Mellinghoff, Paul S Mischel, Thomas G Graeber. Glucose deprivation
activates a metabolic and signaling amplification loop leading to cell death.
Molecular Systems Biology, 2012

Is there a role for carbohydrate restriction in the treatment and prevention of cancer? Rainer J Klement and Ulrike Kämmerer; Nutr Metab (Lond). 2011; 8: 75; Published online 2011 October 26

Brewer, A. Keith Ph.D The High ph Therapy for Cancer, Tests on Mice and Humans Pharmacology Biochemistry & Behavior v. 21, supp 1 pg. 15, 1984

Ambrosone CB, Tang L. Cruciferous vegetable intake and cancer prevention: role of nutrigenetics. Cancer Prev Res (Phila Pa). 2009 Apr;2(4):298-300. 2009.

Angeloni C, Leoncini E, Malaguti M, et al. Modulation of phase II enzymes by sulforaphane: implications for its cardioprotective potential. J Agric Food Chem. 2009 Jun 24;57(12):5615-22. 2009.

Antosiewicz J, Ziolkowski W, Kar S et al. Role of reactive oxygen intermediates in cellular responses to dietary cancer chemopreventive agents. Planta Med. 2008 Oct;74(13):1570-9. 2008.

Banerjee S, Wang Z, Kong D, et al. 3,3'-Diindolylmethane enhances chemosensitivity of multiple chemotherapeutic agents in pancreatic cancer. 3,3'-Diindolylmethane enhances chemosensitivity of multiple chemotherapeutic agents in pancreatic cancer. 2009.

Bhattacharya A, Tang L, Li Y, et al. Inhibition of bladder cancer development by allyl isothiocyanate. Carcinogenesis. 2010 Feb;31(2):281-6. 2010.

Brat P, George S, Bellamy A, et al. Daily Polyphenol Intake in France from Fruit and Vegetables. J. Nutr. 136:2368-2373, September 2006. 2006.

Bryant CS, Kumar S, Chamala S, et al. Sulforaphane induces cell cycle arrest by protecting RB-E2F-1 complex in epithelial ovarian cancer cells. Molecular Cancer 2010, 9:47. 2010.

Carpenter CL, Yu MC, and London SJ. Dietary isothiocyanates, glutathione S-transferase M1 (GSTM1), and lung cancer risk in African Americans and Caucasians from Los Angeles County, California. Nutr Cancer. 2009;61(4):492-9. 2009.

Christopher B, Sanjeez K, Sreedhar C, et al. Sulforaphane induces cell cycle arrest by protecting RB-E2F-1 complex in epithelial ovarian cancer cells. Molecular Cancer Year: 2010 Vol: 9 Issue: 1 Pages/record No.: 47. 2010.

Clarke JD, Dashwood RH, Ho E. Multi-targeted prevention of cancer by sulforaphane. Cancer Lett. 2008 Oct 8;269 (2):291-304. 2008.

Cornelis MC, El-Sohemy A, Campos H. GSTT1 genotype modifies the association between cruciferous vegetable intake and the risk of myocardial infarction. Am J Clin Nutr. 2007 Sep;86(3):752-8. 2007.

Fowke JH, Morrow JD, Motley S, et al. Brassica vegetable consumption reduces urinary F2-isoprostane levels independent of micronutrient intake. Carcinogenesis, October 1, 2006; 27(10): 2096 - 2102. 2006.

Higdon JV, Delage B, Williams DE, et al. Cruciferous Vegetables and Human Cancer Risk: Epidemiologic Evidence and Mechanistic Basis. Pharmacol Res. 2007 March; 55(3): 224-236. 2007.

Hoelzl C, Glatt H, Simic T, et al. DNA protective effects of Brussels sprouts: Results of a human intervention study. AACR Meeting Abstracts, Dec 2007; 2007: B67. 2007.

Hu J, Straub J, Xiao D, et al. Phenethyl isothiocyanate, a cancer chemopreventive constituent of cruciferous vegetables, inhibits cap-dependent translation by regulating the level and phosphorylation of 4E-BP1. Cancer Res. 2007 Apr 15;67(8):3569-73. 2007.

Hutzen B, Willis W, Jones S, et al. Dietary agent, benzyl isothiocyanate inhibits signal transducer and activator of transcription 3 phosphorylation and collaborates with sulforaphane in the growth suppression of PANC-1 cancer cells. Cancer Cell International 2009, 9:24. 2009.

Jiang H, Shang X, Wu H, et al. Combination treatment with resveratrol and sulforaphane induces apoptosis in human U251 glioma cells. Neurochem Res. 2010 Jan;35(1):152-61. 2010.

Kahlon TS, Chiu MC, and Chapman MH. Steam cooking significantly improves in vitro bile acid binding of collard greens, kale, mustard greens, broccoli, green bell pepper, and cabbage. Nutr Res. 2008 Jun,28 (6):351-7. 2008.

Kelemen LE, Cerhan JR, Lim U, et al. Vegetables, fruit, and antioxidant-related nutrients and risk of non-Hodgkin lymphoma: a National Cancer Institute-Surveillance, Epidemiology, and End Results population-based case-control study. Am J Clin Nutr. 2006 Jun;83 (6):1401-10. 2006.

Konsue N, Ioannides C. Modulation of carcinogen-metabolising cytochromes P450 in human liver by the chemopreventive phytochemical phenethyl isothiocyanate, a constituent of cruciferous vegetables. Toxicology. 2010 Feb 9;268(3):184-90. 2010.

Kunimasa K, Kobayashi T, Kaji K et al. Antiangiogenic effects of indole-3-carbinol and 3,3'-diindolylmethane are associated with their differential regulation of ERK1/2 and Akt in tube-forming HUVEC. J Nutr. 2010 Jan;140 (1):1-6. 2010.

Lakhan SE, Kirchgessner A, Hofer M. Inflammatory mechanisms in ischemic stroke: therapeutic approaches. Journal of Translational Medicine 2009, 7:97. 2009.

Larsson SC, Andersson SO, Johansson JE, et al. Fruit and vegetable consumption and risk of bladder cancer: a prospective cohort study. Cancer Epidemiol Biomarkers Prev. 2008 Sep;17(9):2519-22. 2008.

Li F, Hullar MAJ, Schwarz Y, et al. Human Gut Bacterial Communities Are Altered by Addition of Cruciferous Vegetables to a Controlled Fruit- and Vegetable-Free Diet. Journal of Nutrition, Vol. 139, No. 9, 1685-1691, September 2009. 2009.

Lin J, Kamat A, Gu J, et al. Dietary intake of vegetables and fruits and the modification effects of GSTM1 and NAT2 genotypes on bladder cancer risk. Cancer Epidemiol Biomarkers Prev. 2009 Jul;18(7):2090-7. 2009.

Machijima Y, Ishikawa C, Sawada S, et al. Anti-adult T-cell leukemia/lymphoma effects of indole-3-carbinol. Retrovirology 2009, 6:7. 2009.

McMillan M, Spinks EA, and Fenwick GR. Preliminary observations on the effect of dietary brussels sprouts on thyroid function. Hum Toxicol. 1986;5(1):15-19. 1986.

Johnson LW, Weinstock RS. The metabolic syndrome: concepts and controversy. *Mayo Clinic Proceedings.* 2006; 81:1615–20.Liese AD, Roach AK, Sparks KC, Marquart L, D'Agostino RB, Jr., Mayer-Davis EJ. Whole-grain intake and insulin sensitivity: the Insulin Resistance Atherosclerosis Study. *American Journal of Clinical Nutrition.* 2003; 78:965–71. Ludwig DS. Clinical update: the low-glycaemic-index diet. *Lancet.* 2007; 369:890–2.

Foster-Powell K, Holt SH, Brand-Miller JC. International table of glycemic index and glycemic load values: 2002. *American Journal of Clinical Nutrition.* 2002; 76:5–56.

Beulens JW, de Bruijne LM, Stolk RP, et al. High dietary glycemic load and glycemic index increase risk of cardiovascular disease among middle-aged women: a population-based follow-up study. *Journal of the American College of Cardiology.* 2007; 50:14–21.

Halton TL, Willett WC, Liu S, et al. Low-carbohydrate-diet score and the risk of coronary heart disease in women. *New England Journal of Medicine*. 2006; 355:1991–2002.

Anderson JW, Randles KM, Kendall CW, Jenkins DJ. Carbohydrate and fiber recommendations for individuals with diabetes: a quantitative assessment and meta-analysis of the evidence. *Journal of the American College of Nutrition*. 2004; 23:5–17.

Ebbeling CB, Leidig MM, Feldman HA, Lovesky MM, Ludwig DS. Effects of a low-glycemic load vs low-fat diet in obese young adults: a randomized trial. *JAMA*. 2007; 297:2092–102.

Maki KC, Rains TM, Kaden VN, Raneri KR, Davidson MH. Effects of a reduced-glycemic-load diet on body weight, body composition, and cardiovascular disease risk markers in overweight and obese adults. *American Journal of Clinical Nutrition*. 2007; 85:724–34.

Chiu CJ, Hubbard LD, Armstrong J, et al. Dietary glycemic index and carbohydrate in relation to early age-related macular degeneration. *American Journal of Clinical Nutrition*. 2006; 83:880–6.

Chavarro JE, Rich-Edwards JW, Rosner BA, Willett WC. A prospective study of dietary carbohydrate quantity and quality in relation to risk of ovulatory infertility. *European Journal of Clinical Nutrition*. 2007.

Higginbotham S, Zhang ZF, Lee IM et al. Dietary glycemic load and risk of colorectal cancer in the Women's Health Study. *J Natl Cancer Inst*. 2004; 96:229-33.

Liu S, Willett WC. Dietary glycemic load and atherothrombotic risk. *Curr Atheroscler Rep*. 2002; 4:454–61.

Willett W, Manson J, Liu S. Glycemic index, glycemic load, and risk of type 2 diabetes. *American Journal of Clinical Nutrition*. 2002; 76:274S–80S.

Foster GD, Wyatt HR, Hill JO, et al. A randomized trial of a low-carbohydrate diet for obesity. *New England Journal of Medicine*. 2003; 348:2082–90.

Samaha FF, Iqbal N, Seshadri P, et al. A low-carbohydrate as compared with a low-fat diet in severe obesity. *New England Journal of Medicine*. 2003; 348:2074–81.

Gardner CD, Kiazand A, Alhassan S, et al. Comparison of the Atkins, Zone, Ornish, and LEARN diets for change in weight and related risk factors among overweight premenopausal women: the A TO Z Weight Loss Study: a randomized trial. *JAMA*. 2007; 297:969–77.Halton TL, Liu S, Manson JE, Hu FB. Low-carbohydrate-diet score and risk of type 2 diabetes in women. *Am J Clin Nutr*. 2008;87:339-46.

Sacks FM, Bray GA, Carey VJ, et al. Comparison of Weight-Loss Diets with Different Compositions of Fat, Protein, and Carbohydrates. *N Engl J Med*. 2009; 360:859-873.

Moore LE, Brennan P, Karami S, et al. Glutathione S-transferase polymorphisms, cruciferous vegetable intake and cancer risk in the Central and Eastern European Kidney Cancer Study. Carcinogenesis. 2007 Sep;28(9):1960-4. Epub 2007 Jul 7. 2007.

Nettleton JA, Steffen LM, Mayer-Davis EJ, et al. Dietary patterns are associated with biochemical markers of inflammation and endothelial activation in the Multi-Ethnic Study of Atherosclerosis (MESA). Am J Clin Nutr. 2006 Jun;83(6):1369-79. 2006.

Rungapamestry V, Duncan AJ, Fuller Z et al. Effect of cooking brassica vegetables on the subsequent hydrolysis and metabolic fate of glucosinolates. Proc Nutr Soc. 2007 Feb;66(1):69-81. 2007.

Silberstein JL, Parsons JK. Evidence-based principles of bladder cancer and diet. Urology. 2010 Feb;75(2):340-6. 2010.

Steinbrecher A, Linseisen J. Dietary Intake of Individual Glucosinolates in Participants of the EPIC-Heidelberg Cohort Study. Ann Nutr Metab 2009;54:87-96. 2009.

Way TD, Kao MC, Lin JK. Apigenin induces apoptosis through proteasomal degradation of HER2/neu in HER2/neu-overexpressing breast cancer cells via the phosphatidylinositol-3'-kinase/Akt-dependent pathway. J Biol Chem. 2004;279:4479–4489. PubMed

Birt DF, Mitchell D, Gold B, Pour P, Pinch HC. Inhibition of ultraviolet light induced skin carcinogenesis in SKH-1 mice by apigenin, a plant flavonoid. Anticancer Res. 1997;17:85–91. PubMed

Patel D, Shukla S, Gupta S. Apigenin and cancer chemoprevention: progress, potential and promise. Int J Oncol. 2007;30:233–245. PubMed

Gates MA, Tworoger SS, Hecht JL, De Vivo I, Rosner B, Hankinson SE. A prospective study of dietary flavonoid intake and incidence of epithelial ovarian cancer. Int. J Cancer. 2007;121:2225–223. PubMed

Shukla S, Mishra A, Fu P, MacLennan GT, Resnick MI, Gupta S. Up-regulation of insulin-like growth factor binding protein-3 by apigenin leads to growth inhibition and apoptosis of 22Rv1 xenograft in athymic nude mice. FASEB J. 2005;19:2042–2044. PubMed

Tang L, Zirpoli GR, Guru K, et al. Consumption of Raw Cruciferous Vegetables is Inversely Associated with Bladder Cancer Risk. 2007 Apr 15;67(8):3569-73. 2007.

Tang L, Zirpoli GR, Jayaprakash V, et al. Cruciferous vegetable intake is inversely associated with lung cancer risk among smokers: a case-control study. BMC Cancer 2010, 10:162. 2010.

Tarozzi A, Morroni F, Merlicco A, et al. Sulforaphane as an inducer of glutathione prevents oxidative stress-induced cell death in a dopaminergic-like neuroblastoma cell line. J Neurochem. 2009 Dec;111(5):1161-71. 2009.

Thompson CA, Habermann TM, Wang AH, et al. Antioxidant intake from fruits, vegetables and other sources and risk of non-Hodgkin's lymphoma: the Iowa Women's Health Study. Int J Cancer. 2010 Feb 15;126(4):992-1003. 2010.

Zhang Y. Allyl isothiocyanate as a cancer chemopreventive phytochemical. Mol Nutr Food Res. 2010 Jan;54(1):127-35. 2010.

46672644R00144

Made in the USA
San Bernardino, CA
07 August 2019